Building Blocks of Nutrition for Bodybuilders

By: Jeffrey Bedeaux

Table of Contents

Whole food vs. protein drinks

Main points for building muscle

Keep volume low and intensity high

Train briefly and infrequently

Train for strength

Use an appropriate repetition range

Focus on the major muscle groups

Use proper training style and technique

Emphasize recovery more than you think you should

Eat well and often

Combine machines and free weights

Keep a daily workout record

Diet to obtain muscular definition and low bodyfat

Questions and answers

Introduction

About this book

Hello and welcome! Thanks for purchasing my new e-book. It's loaded with revolutionary proven knowledge and techniques that will allow you to quickly and efficiently transform your body to whatever level of fitness and muscularity you desire. You can do muscle toning or firming or conditioning for a sport or **even adding 20, 40, 60 pounds of new, hard muscle** to your frame. All without drugs and without spending a fortune on nutritional supplements and without wasting your time in the gym.

You see, a while ago my 25-year-old friend told me was getting into lifting weights at the gym and he wanted to know what I thought he should be doing in the gym to maximize his results. He knew that I wrote books on the subject, performed research on trainees from 16 to 82 years of age, measured the results every step of the way and synthesized them into full workouts and specialization workouts. He knew all that and more but he didn't want to read that much, he just wanted his best friend to tell him the core knowledge from all those books and all that research. The best of the best without any preamble, padding myself on the back or self-serving BS about how smart I was compared to others. So I gave it to him. Nothing more; nothing less.

That made me realize I really could condense what I've learned developing new data, feedback from customers, and experience from personal consultations. Everything into a book that I could make available to anyone in the world via the Internet.

And that's what you have right now. The best information garnered from years of research in real world testing. I urge you to read every word of it. The knowledge you need is in these pages and is laid out in a concise format and I don't repeat the same things over and over. That is with the exception of safety. Safety is the most important piece of information you can get out of this book. With that said I wouldn't dwell on it too much.

Getting the most from this book

If you are like most guys, you're tempted to turn to the chapters on workouts and dive right into your workouts with those killer techniques and principles. That's because most muscleheads see bodybuilding as merely hoisting weights up-and-down, over and over, slowly increasing the weight, under some misguided concept of this is what builds muscle. These are the guys who are always on the look out for the magic routine that has eluded them for so long. Don't make that mistake!

Now I know you're not going to like to hear this, but read this manual all the way through before beginning your program. I want you to get on the gym floor in the quickest time possible but I want you to be armed with the advanced knowledge needed to put that time to good use. If you skip a chapter thinking you already know everything needed to know about that training factor, you could be setting yourself up for a big disappointment. But don't worry I'll be there every step of the way.

We will be covering a lot of information in this book. Information that is anything but common knowledge even among the professional bodybuilders who rely on anabolic steroids for their massive gains. Well, there you have it. I've sufficiently warned you of the dangers of skipping ahead in this book and I've given you a couple of "extra emphasis" tools to make sure you get the most important details from all information I have jammed into these pages.

Also, you will notice a couple of inches of open space at the bottom of each page; I did this for a reason. I want you to write down and highlight the most important parts for you. This open space is for your notes. By reading and writing the ideas that really connect with you, you will be able to absorb and use those points without even being aware of it. Print out this book and write all over it; I want you to squeeze every benefit out of the huge amount of information within these pages.

Two other tools you will see throughout this book that will help you understand the key points are _The Doctor Says_ dialog box and the _Doctor's Prescription_ dialog box. Look for boxes like these as you are reading:

> The Doctor Says:
> "Look here for insights into the topic being discussed."

> Doctor's Prescription:
> Look in these boxes for action steps you can take.

These 2 dialog boxes will help you get the most important information first. Also use them as a guideline for writing your own notes at the bottom of each page. After you have read this book you can skim through it later and read only the dialog boxes and your personal notes to re-connect with all the information contained in this book. I have found this technique to be very valuable to me when I want to skim a book I have already read and review the key points.

So here's what I want you to do now. If you have already been busting your ass in the gym training three to four days or more per week. Take a week off! You'll understand why later, but for now just plan on using that week to review this manual and fully prepare for your fiery return. If you're relatively new to bodybuilding, or it has been awhile since you've been in the gym, take the next week to introduce your body to what it's about to experience. In order to avoid overloading your body to the point of shutdown it's wise to begin a light exercise routine to prepare your muscles, joints and ligaments for the upcoming barrage. You don't want to go all out to the point you can barely move the next day. That would defeat the whole purpose of the first couple weeks of this program. Besides if you're looking for is an intense workout session, the real workout is coming up.

Dedication

This book is dedicated to every bodybuilder and athlete who has an acquiring rational mind; to every person who can throw off the chains of comfortable habit and unproven premises and move into new direction that is guided by reason and observational evidence, no matter where that direction takes him; to every person to try something immediately and thinks "How can I make this better?" To every person who is unafraid to challenge the false beliefs of the herd and lead others out of the cave and into the light.

In the world of bodybuilding it is these people with these genetics who are truly the greatest champions of the human race. To these people not just in the science of human strength but also in every science we all owe our enormous gratitude.

<u>Why an e-book?</u>

Some people ask me why I wrote this as an e-book. I could have written the draft of this book and taken to a mainstream book publisher, but there are a few reasons why I self-published this as an e-book and they all benefit you.

Freedom of content: E-books can contain links to related material, special pages or even built-in programs. Also big publishing companies don't like controversy. They don't like writers being too blunt about certain topics. They prefer to re-edit or re-word certain things. With an e-book, which I both write and publish, I conclude whatever content I want to include. Which leads me to…

Freedom of style: Any writer does better when he uses his own "voice". For example, in a mainstream publication I would have to say, "many professional bodybuilders use dangerous drugs to augment their muscular development." But in my own e-book I can say, "pro bodybuilding is filled with unbridled use of every type of drug imaginable.

Steroids represent less than 10 percent of what drugs bodybuilders actually use today. The full truth is that they use up to 20 prescription drugs at the same time and 1000% of the recommended safe dose. They take drugs intended for diabetes, cancer, dwarfism, pain, bloating, cardiology, hematology, impotence; the list goes on and on.

Athletes and regular folks are dropping dead every year and the huge meltdown is coming because the real health effects (tumors, heart failure, kidney failure, etc) appear to take at least fifteen years to show up. Soon we'll be hearing about the failing health of the great names of bodybuilding from the '80s and '90s, if you haven't heard already." Try finding that kind of plain talk in a nice mainstream book. I'm sure you won't find it especially if the author puts down supplements anyway since that's where the real cash cow is in bodybuilding.

Freedom from templates: Mainstream publishers have a formula they have to follow. It is just the realities of the book business. Right now is the larger book format (9" x 11") with approximately 220 pages; it is all about shelf space in the bookstores and perceived value. So a new e-book with about 120 pages loaded with new ideas that's guaranteed to put 40 pounds of muscle on you doesn't have a prayer of getting into print, but a 220 page book showing women doing "workouts" with 3 pound dumbbells gets in every bookstore and featured every woman's magazine.

The perception of what is valuable is very different from what really has value in the gym. An e-book format allows me to get right to the point without adding a bunch of filler, such as lots and lots of pictures that you have already seen, to get the book up to 220 pages.

The amount of information packed into this e-book took 17 years to determine and compile. It can unlock the greatest muscle growth you've ever experienced. When Einstein writes $E=MC^2$ on a piece of paper, it doesn't take a many pages but that knowledge can unlock enormous power.

Freedom of marketing: Digital content and the Internet is the wave of the future in publishing. When a mainstream book is published it gets an initial marketing push by the publisher and then it's all done. E-books can be promoted by links, banners, affiliate programs, and "word of mouse" that keep it in front of bodybuilders every day. Why should you care about that? The financial success of this e-book fuels the next one and that brings you more useful research information instead of the crap that's available in many books. As you can see in the bookstores, mainstream publishers say the same thing day after day, year after year.

Freedom of access: Less than 5% of the world's population lives in America. It can be pretty difficult and expensive to get an American book delivered to Turkey. But an e-book can be delivered around the world without extra costs and you can be reading it 20 seconds after you buy it.

And I'm not talking hypothetically here; this e-book not only sold copies in the United States and Canada, it also sold in the United Kingdom, France, Germany, Sweden, Switzerland, Australia, Brazil, Ireland, Singapore, South Africa, Denmark, Malaysia, China, Japan, Belarus, American Samoa and the Netherlands. All in the first 60 days!

Like the bodybuilders in the above countries around the world you're about to discover this e-book is absolutely loaded with useful information you can apply in your next workout. You're literally minutes away from the most productive workouts of your life.

<u>**Why I wrote this book**</u>

First let me explain why I wrote this book, I'll phrase it into a short story were I'm sure you can identify with the main character.

Let me introduce you to Average Joe. Joe is very typical of the bodybuilders trying to pack on muscle in today's gyms. Determined to look like "the huge guys" in the magazines, he signed up for his membership at the local gym, buys his weightlifting gloves and belt and all the other "essential tools" for packing on the pounds, and begins his quest.

At the gym he follows the lead of all the other "muscleheads" and begins bench pressing, curling, and squatting the most weight he can. Like the other misinformed Joes, he thinks that working harder and harder, steadily increasing the weight on the bar will force his body into growth beyond his wildest dreams. He makes some gains; enough to keep pushing on but soon finds himself stagnated.

Not seeing any more strength or size development Joe decides to go to the next level. He looks around the gym for the biggest iron pumping "consultant" he can find that also looks friendly enough to talk to. That guy is The Juice. Joe approaches Juice to inquire about the secrets to his bodybuilding. Juice tells Joe everything he knows about what exercises to choose, how much weight to use, what to eat and what "super supplements" to use.

Joe sets out again following everything Juice tells him; positive he now has the missing links to maximum growth. Some of what Juice told Joe was enough to move him out of his plateau temporarily. Within a few weeks he finds his strength and size stalemated again.

Frustrated Joe decides to turn to the "experts". He goes to the local bookstore and picks up every bodybuilding magazine they have and begins his research. Obviously with arms and legs the size of telephone poles and a chest the size of 2 Webster's dictionaries, anything these pros have to say must be gospel. Then there all the ads for the top-secret supplement discoveries promising you God-like powers from all the "latest" scientific research.

Confused and frustrated Joe spent a small fortune on supplements and is back in the gym. He is loaded with tips from all the pros and has so many "secret potions" running through his veins that he can be declared off-limits as a toxic waste dump! He makes a small gain, only to find it wither away as he hits "the wall". The wall is the place that all beginning and novice bodybuilders hit when they realize that building muscle is a whole lot harder than those hulking professionals in the magazines make it look.

Now comes the moment of truth. Here are the facts.

Fact: All those pro bodybuilders trying to coax you to purchase the next wave of natural supplements guaranteeing massive growth, got that big not from the natural supplements they are marketing but rather by pumping massive quantities of anabolic steroids into their veins.

Fact: The killer pre-contest and mass building routines those pros let you in on are enough to throw any bodybuilder into chronic overtraining without the aid of a serious dose of dangerous growth hormone and steroids. Or make you sick from a depressed immune system or seriously injure yourself.

Fact: The bodybuilding supplement market is a multi-multi-million dollar industry that is supported by well-intentioned serious seekers of muscle and fitness such as yourself, fall prey to the ads and articles designed for one thing, to take your hard earned money.

Fact: Supplement manufacturers and gym owners all follow the six-month rule of marketing. Basically six months is how long research has shown it takes the average "seeker of strength" to join a gym, purchase the supplements they're convinced they need, reach the wall where they see no more gains, get frustrated, and quit their workout program.

Fact: Those same bodybuilding magazines that projected air of "objectivity" actually own many of the supplements they're advertising and are recommending in their magazines.

Here are some of the worst offenders:

Flex — Weider Supplements
Muscle & Fitness — Weider Supplements
MuscleMag — Muscle Tech
Muscular Development — Twinlab
Muscle Media — EAS

These companies weren't stupid. They realized early on that they could sell you a magazine full of great looking perfectly sculpted columns of muscle to make you feel puny and weak; then offer you ad after ad of expensive supplements with pumped up scientific claims to milk you for even more of your dough.

<u>Be careful</u>

Caution: This program involves a systemic progression of muscular overload that leads to lifting extremely heavy weights. As a result, a proper warm-up of muscles, tendons, ligaments, and joints is mandatory at beginning of every workout.

Warning: As this is a very intense program, it requires both a thorough knowledge of proper exercise form and a base level of strength fitness. Although exercise is very beneficial, the potential does exist for injury, especially if the trainee is not in good physical condition. As always consult with your physician before beginning any program of progressive weight training or exercise. If you feel any strain or pain when you start exercising, stop immediately and consult your physician.

The building blocks

I believe many of us make the process of bodybuilding far more complicated than it needs to be. This is especially true when it comes to nutrition. I've come to this conclusion after answering literally thousands of questions from bodybuilders for years. Through seminars, letters, phone consultations, and contact through the Internet, the same questions were asked and the same challenges were encountered over and over again. It didn't matter what level of experience, number of accomplishments, individual circumstances, or what part of the world a bodybuilder lived, when it comes to nutrition, our patterns of thinking and the obstacles they faced were basically the same.

As I strive to strengthen my skills as an effective bodybuilding coach, one of my goals is to simplify the bodybuilding process. The bottom line is that **we are all after the same things; to build muscle, lose body fat, or a combination** of building muscle and losing body fat. We also want to do so in the most efficient ways and in the shortest period of time.

If you embrace the nutritional strategies I've outlined in this book, how you need to build muscle and lose body fat will be simpler. **Notice the word I used was** *simple*—**not easy!** Nothing is easy; nothing worth having, anyway. Eating to create a lean and muscular physique is no exception.

Why you need good nutrition

If you want to produce high-quality muscle and maintain lower body fat levels from the time and effort you invest in training, you *must* feed yourself properly. Many experts feel the way you eat accounts for as much as 50 percent of the way you look. If you want an impressive muscular body, you are going to have to pay close attention to what you are eating.

Sound nutrition is that important to your bodybuilding efforts. A heavy emphasis needs to be placed on studying winning nutritional strategies and executing those strategies on a consistent basis.

Motivation builds the foundation of good eating habits

"I'm so confused about nutrition!" many bodybuilders often complain. "My training is great but, when it comes to how I should eat, I don't have a clue!"

Good eating habits are built upon a foundation of motivation. Let's get honest with ourselves for a moment. Is the difficulty in this particular situation in *understanding* nutrition? Or, is the real challenge *following through* with eating the way we already know we should?

Let's admit what's really going on in some of our minds. Eating delicious foods is one of life's simplest, easiest-to-attain, and greatest pleasures. Sometimes, it's very difficult to stay away from food that doesn't support our bodybuilding efforts. Great-tasting and unhealthy food becomes too much of a temptation for us. Even when we are committed to eating properly, it's sometimes too difficult to break away from our busy schedules and eat our meals at all; whether they are good for us or not.

The key to eating to build muscle comes down to being properly motivated to do so. Because you are taking the time to read this nutritional advice, I assume you're pretty motivated. This is a great time to determine exactly why *today* is the day you'll make the commitment to earn the physique you really want by eating right. If you know *why* you want to do something, figuring out *how* to do it will become much easier. You must first take care of figuring out *why* and, hopefully, my advice will help you figure out *how* to meet your physique enhancing goals.

Eating to build muscle and lose body fat is a *way of thinking* just as much as it is a series of actions. Many bodybuilders get easily confused, frustrated, and eventually overwhelmed with the subject of proper nutrition. Rock-solid bodybuilding nutrition doesn't need to be complicated in order to be effective.

Three important keys to understanding effective nutrition

Let's break down and simplify this important aspect of bodybuilding. You basically need to understand three things about nutrition:

1. The main purpose for each of the three macronutrients: Protein, carbohydrates, and fat

2. The "right" ratio, or the "correct" percentages, of protein, carbohydrates, and fat that your food should be divided into in order to meet your bodybuilding goals

3. The number of calories you should consume to meet your specific physique-enhancement goals

Good nutrition seems much easier when it is broken down and you look it at from that perspective, doesn't it? But what do the three macronutrients do for our bodies? What ratio of our food should be allocated to protein, carbohydrates, and fat? How do I determine how many calories I should eat? I'll answer those questions—and a whole lot more.

Those questions about nutrition provide a wide range of answers that are not necessarily easy to find. Unfortunately, there are no easier ways around this fact. There are no magic numbers, solutions, or formulas that I, nor anyone else, can give you to make the process effortless; no matter what you are told. These answers not only vary from person to person, they also can vary within the very same *person* during different periods of time.

With simplicity and efficiency in mind, let's discuss the macronutrients. In general terms, all food is broken down into three major groups of macronutrients; protein, carbohydrates, and fat. Here is a simple explanation of what they are and what each of them does for our bodies:

Protein, your #1 priority

Protein, far and away, is the most important nutrient you'll need to build muscle on your body. **Muscle *is* protein. Protein *is* muscle.** Without enough protein, you'll have a very difficult time seeing results from your training. Plain and simple, you're simply not going to grow muscle without a sufficient amount of protein.

It is important for you to maintain a balance in the positive flow of nitrogen on a consistent basis. By this, I mean you absolutely *must* consume more nitrogen than you excrete. You need to keep your body in a positive protein accrual environment. If you happen to be excreting more nitrogen than you consume, it doesn't matter. I have discovered, like many other bodybuilders, the more protein I consume the bigger and stronger I get.

How much protein should I eat to build muscle?

How much is the "right" amount of protein to eat each day, you ask? 100 grams? 250 grams? 500 grams? You will need to *experiment* to determine what the proper amount of protein is that will keep you in a positive protein accrual environment.

Bodybuilders should start with a gram per pound of bodyweight—and move *upwards* from there. Many experts estimate this is how much the average hard-training bodybuilder needs per day. My only suggestion would be, if your body can efficiently use more, then by all means, give it more and build more muscle!

> The Doctor Says:
> Protein is the most important piece of your nutrition program. Always have some protein in each meal so you will have a constant flow of amino acids in your system. This alone will help you keep your hard earned muscle while at the same time you can add on more mass.

There is also a very old, outdated, and conservative method of determining the "proper" amount of protein you should ingest. Unfortunately, too many bodybuilders hold on tightly to this theory. I don't believe there is any way possible this cookie cutter rule can apply to everyone; especially every single hard-training bodybuilder. This method suggests that you multiply your body weight in kilograms times 1.5 to figure the grams of protein to consume daily. FYI - divide your weight in pounds by 2.2 to determine how much you weigh in kilograms.

The only reason I even include this guideline is because 9 out of 10 people in the bodybuilding world are going to tell you this is the "right" amount of protein; not a single gram more! If you ingest any more protein than that, they warn, you are going to damage your kidneys.

I suggest you shouldn't be so conservative about your protein consumption; especially if you want to make the most use of your hard training and pack on some serious, rock-solid muscle mass! But, if you do try this widely accepted formula, be sure to experiment upwards from there. If you are able to handle more than that amount efficiently, you will probably gain more muscle. One thing you don't want to do is rob yourself of even one more ounce of precious muscle!

"How much protein should I eat then? I calculate my total should be 177 grams a day." Bodybuilder A says. I recommend determining the amount of protein you should eat a little differently. Instead of figuring out the total grams of protein you can efficiently digest in the entire day; **determine how much you can efficiently digest at each meal.**

Why? If you eat your daily total, let's say, of 300 grams of protein in *four* meals as opposed to 7, the efficiency of how your body digests that protein would differ, wouldn't it?

If you take those 300 grams of protein and divide that total by four meals, that would equal 75 grams per meal. Those 300 grams of protein divided by 7 meals equals 43 grams per meal. Obviously, your body will have a much easier time digesting the 43 grams per meal than it would 75 grams. You are eating the very same amount of protein for the entire day—but are creating a big difference in the efficiency of its digestion and utilization. **Your body would have a much easier time using the protein to help build muscle if it was spaced out evenly throughout the day.**

Let me ask you a question: Are you confused about the amount of protein some experts in the bodybuilding community are recommending? You really should be more concerned with consistently eating more frequent, high-protein meals and properly spacing them throughout your day. The average meal replacement contains about 40 grams of protein. Even those people who don't think the human body can assimilate large amounts of protein will agree that it can digest 40 grams every two to three hours, right?

Every two to three hours creates what I call a **"Protein Window of Opportunity."** The more of these opportunities you take advantage of; the more you will augment your efforts in the gym. The more you consume high-quality protein during these windows—regardless of the amount of protein in that "window" or daily total of protein you think your body needs—the more muscle you will build. The key to successfully building muscle is eating smaller, more frequent meals throughout the day. Instead of worrying about that often-debated daily total of protein, break it down into two-hour to three-hour increments.

> Doctor's Prescription:
> Space out your protein consumption throughout the day to allow your body to assimilate as much protein as possible. This way you won't be sending your protein (and hard earned cash) right down the toilet.

Do the math. The guy who eats 7 meals as opposed to four meals a day has almost twice as many "Protein Windows of Opportunity" to take advantage of. Four a day, times seven days a week, equals 21 more "windows." Every month that's 91 more and every year the total grows to an incredible 1,092 more "Protein Windows of Opportunity" that are used. All other factors being the same, who do you think will build more muscle over the course of that year?

Good protein sources

Food	Serving Size	Calories	Protein (g)	% cal. from protein
Whey protein	1 scoop	100	24	96
Egg whites	6	102	24	95
Turkey breast	6 oz.	180	40	89
Tuna	6 oz.	180	39	87
Ground turkey	6 oz.	220	48	87
Chicken breast	6 oz.	180	36	80
Sirloin steak	6 oz.	345	51	59
Chicken thigh	6 oz.	330	36	51
Lean ground beef	6 oz.	435	45	43
Pork	6 oz.	315	24	31
Ground beef	6 oz.	270	15	23
Salmon	6 oz.	300	42	56
Eggs	1	75	6	34
Peanuts	1 oz.	90	4	18
Yogurt	8 oz.	120	13	43
Skim milk	8 oz.	90	9	40
Swiss cheese	1 oz.	90	8	35
2% milk	8 oz.	120	8	27
cheddar cheese	1 oz.	110	7	25
Whole milk	8 oz.	150	8	21

The danger of eating too much protein

Is eating too much protein dangerous? Many experts will tell you that eating too much protein will cause damage to your kidneys. Obviously, by the amount of protein I've been eating consistently every single day throughout my life, I either don't believe this is true or I am willing to take the risk in order to reach my ambitious bodybuilding goals. Besides, according to medical journals, you would have to eat 600+ grams of protein per day for a long time to have an effect on your kidneys.

Do I think, regardless of what the experts say you should ingest a large amount of protein like I choose to do? I can't make that decision for you. I can, however, share with you the reason why I do despite some people's warnings. The people that I trust to give me accurate information tell me there are no scientific studies to back up those doom-and-gloom claims. They have theorized that the experts have come to their conclusion because the kidneys play a major role in the synthesizing of protein. Thus, if they are forced to do more work than the average person, they are at a greater risk to suffer damage.

I, myself, haven't had any problems. I always make sure I do the things doctors recommend to help your body digest the protein like drinking a lot of water.

I am certain, however, that I have built a significant amount of muscle mass every single year that I've been training. I attribute much of that to **consistently eating high-quality protein** day after day, week after week, month after month, and year after year.

I firmly believe my body is able to assimilate most of the 300 grams I eat every day. There are studies that suggest the **hard training athletes can efficiently assimilate up to a whopping 72 grams of protein at a time.** That's far more than the old "multiply your body weight in kilograms times 1.5" formula!

I choose to take my chances, but you should talk to your physician if you have any concerns about eating excessive amounts of protein. I don't know anything about the effects of "excess" protein for certain. You'll need to make the decision of exactly how much protein to eat for yourself.

Carbohydrates, the energy you need

Carbohydrates give you the energy to train hard in the gym and carry out your everyday activities. Your body needs carbohydrates on a consistent basis throughout the day to feed the brain, which uses glucose, or blood sugar, as its primary energy source. Glucose is a carbohydrate used by every cell in the body as fuel.

When carbohydrates stored in the body are depleted too far, the body will convert precious muscle-building protein into glucose instead of regular carbohydrates to give the body the energy it needs. As a bodybuilder, you want to do everything you possibly can to avoid this from occurring. The very last thing you want is to have your hard-earned muscle mass sacrificed for energy. Consuming enough carbohydrates will prevent this from happening.

Excess carbohydrates, however, will be converted into fat. How can you avoid eating too many carbohydrates? I was once offered a suggestion I found to be very helpful. The strategy was to **eat the majority of carbohydrates in the morning and immediately after working out.** These are ideal times for the body to process carbohydrates more rapidly.

Some people believe you should limit your carbohydrate consumption after 6 or 7 p.m. They believe carbohydrates are converted to body fat much easier at that time because of your body's ability to burn fat is reduced while sleeping. Others have a different opinion. They believe it doesn't matter when you eat your carbohydrates. The body processes carbohydrates the same all the time.

> The Doctor Says:
> You will need to experiment with your carb consumption. Everybody is different so there isn't a cookie cutter program that will work for everyone. It goes without saying but, experiment with the healthy carbohydrates; we all know what a candy bar will do (or not do) for your training.

Personally, I agree with the latter opinion. Carbohydrates in the morning, carbohydrates in the evening, or carbohydrates in the afternoon, in my opinion, it ultimately doesn't matter when you eat them. What is important is, at the end of the day, the calories that you've burned are greater than the calories you've consumed.

How do you determine the "right" amount of carbohydrates you should eat? I decide the amount of carbohydrates I'll eat this way:

As a bodybuilder, I will *always* keep my protein intake high to build muscle (usually, this is about 300 grams a day). If I'm trying to get lean or stay lean, I will closely monitor the fat in my diet. I also realize I must stay within a certain calorie range to meet my personal goals. What's left to consider? Only carbohydrates. I eat enough carbohydrates to give me just enough energy to train heavy and with intensity, have enough energy to do my regular life's activities, and to manage my body fat level. After I total the calories from my essential protein and incidental fat, the calories coming from carbohydrates can't cause me to exceed the total calories I've allotted myself for the day. The calories derived from carbohydrates must "sandwich" in between.

Starchy carbohydrates, stay away from them

As I work with more bodybuilders from around the world, I'm beginning to realize the biggest problem for most of us is over eating starchy or grainy carbohydrates. I think the biggest problem with starchy, complex carbohydrates is that they are very easy to overeat. It doesn't take very much rice or pasta to add up to a lot of calories.

You don't get very much food in a single serving of starchy carbohydrates; especially for the amount of calories that one serving contains. One serving of white rice contains about 150 calories and about 35 grams of carbohydrates. One serving of rice adds up to a puny 3/4 of a cup—and that's after it's cooked! That's not very much food.

How often do you stop after eating only 3/4 of a cup of cooked white rice when you are hungry, really? "Whoops, I guess I put a little too much in that measuring cup. Oh well." I know how it goes; I've been there too! I think the reason why a lot of bodybuilders who eat "clean" but can't get lean as quickly as they want or even stay fat is because they're unaware of overeating starchy carbohydrates.

I tend to lose body fat more quickly when I avoid starchy carbohydrates altogether. I believe the reason why is because I ingest fewer *calories* by replacing them with vegetables, or fibrous carbohydrates. You can eat an entire 16-ounce bag of broccoli has only 175 calories and 20 grams of carbohydrates.

I used to believe avoiding carbohydrates like rice, potatoes, oatmeal, and pasta and substituting them for vegetables was better for fat loss because I thought different types carbohydrates were digested a lot differently. I now feel that it's all a matter of calories burned versus calories ingested. That's how you effectively lose body fat. It doesn't matter which kind of carbohydrates you eat.

> Doctor's Prescription:
> Research the foods you eat. Buy a book or scan the internet to get the breakdown of the foods that make up your individual diet. This way you will know what adjustments to make.

You should get your hands on a calorie-conversion book and look up just exactly what is considered a serving of your favorite carbohydrate, and more importantly, exactly how many calories that serving contains. In many cases, you'll be surprised just how small the serving is and how large the number of calories it contains. When dieting strictly, what type of foods do you crave the most and find the most satisfying? If you are like me, it's definitely complex carbohydrates!

Choose the right carbs at the right time

Slow-digesting carbs: You will want to use slow-digesting carbs for a large portion of your carb intake since they give you a slow and steady supply of energy. They also maintain a steady release of insulin which aids in the control of bodyfat levels.

Good selections of slow-digesting carbs:

Apples
Beans
Brown rice
Cream of rye cereal
Oatmeal
Oat bran cereal
Oranges
Red potatoes
Rye bread
Seven-grain bread
Yogurt

Medium-digesting carbs: You should also make medium-digesting carbs a big part of your diet. They are called the "in-between-carbs" since they neither shoot into the bloodstream nor trickle in the way slow-digesting carbs do. Starchy carbs, which make up most of the calories eaten by people, also fall into this category.

Good selections of medium-digesting carbs:

Buckwheat pancakes
Corn
Most fruit
Honey
Peas
White rice
Most pasta
Yams

Fast-digesting-carbs: Sugar and other simple carbs fit into this category because they hit the bloodstream rapidly. They are most helpful after training when your muscles are starving for nutrients and need energy ASAP. Throughout the rest of the day it is a good idea to keep your consumption of fast-digesting carbs to a minimum.

Good selections of fast-digesting carbs:

Cold cereals
Cream of rice
Cream of wheat
Gatorade
Potatoes
Pop
White bread
Bagels

Here I'll break down the carb information a little more: These charts will separate carbs by complex, fruit, and vegetable types.

Complex carbs chart

Food	Serving	Carbs (g)
Black beans	3 oz dry	20
Brown rice	1.5 oz dry	20
Multigrain bread	1 slice	20
Oatmeal	3 oz dry	20
Pasta	1 oz dry	20
Pinto beans	2 oz dry	20
Potatoes	4 oz baked	20
White rice	1 oz dry	20

Fruit chart

Food	Serving	Carbs (g)
Apple	1 medium	20
Banana	1 medium	20
Cherries	1 cup	20
Orange	1 medium	20
Peaches	2 medium	20
Pear	1 medium	20
Pineapple	5 oz	20
Watermelon	10 oz	20

Vegetable chart

Food	Serving	Carbs (g)
Broccoli	1 cup	10
Carrots	5 oz	10
Cauliflower	2 cups	10
Green peppers	2 medium	10
Peas	0.5 cup	10
Spinach	1 cup	10
Yellow squash	1 cup	10

Fats, they aren't all bad

Fat in your diet serves a vital purpose for the body. Fat acts as a structural component for all cell membranes and supplies necessary chemical substrates for hormonal production. Fat protects vital organs and carries fat-soluble vitamins. **Your body needs fat so don't try to avoid it completely.** Many experts feel that 10-20 percent of your total dietary calories should come from fat.

Why does every package of cottage cheese, milk, dressing, or yogurt make this huge deal of it's low fat content, usually deceptively advertised as: "98% fat free!" which still could mean that a considerable chunk of the calories from the product comes from fat. Who cares? The words: "Fat Free" sells like crazy.

The reason for this is obvious - we have been in a state of complete media overload, hammered with messages about how bad fats are for us, on a daily basis for many years now. Bodyfat, cardiovascular disease, diabetes…you know the list.

Fat isn't the devil. In fact, you'd get sick, malnourished, and eventually die if it wasn't for the fat in your food. You need it, period. Like with everything else, it's only a matter of keeping things in a proper perspective, and maintain a healthy balance.

One thing that is true about fat is that it is the biggest bandit around when it comes to packing calories. **For every gram of fat you eat, you get more than twice as many calories as a gram of protein or carbs.** Fats have 9 calories per gram as opposed to 4 calories per gram for the others.

You have to look at the big picture when you review your fat intake. What does it consist of? Saturated, unsaturated, or polyunsaturated fat? If there's plenty of the first, and little of the two latter, it's time for you to consider your eating habits. As a rule of thumb, it's the saturated fat that causes most of the trouble for people. Granted - all three categories yield the same number of calories - but they are very different when it comes to what they do once inside your body.

Saturated fats are found in animal sources, such as meat, egg yolks, milk, and peanuts and coconuts. These are the nasty little creeps that clog up your arteries, most readily settle in on your midsection, and generally do their best to mess your health up.

The "good" fats, on the other hand, are found mostly in vegetables and fish. **Olive oil, flax seed oil, and fish oil are prime examples of good sources for "good" fat.** However, make note that we're talking fish oil, not fish **liver** oil here. Fish liver oil may contain massive doses of vitamin A, which is fat-soluble and can be toxic if overdosed. Not cyanide, drop-dead toxic, but the kind of thing that could make you pretty sick and miserable if consistently overdosed over a period of time.

So what are the benefits of fat? For one, we have the essential fatty acids (EFA). As the name implies, these are essential for your survival, just like any vitamin or mineral. In short, they're part of the big puzzle that keeps you alive an' kicking, pal! **Fish oils are generally very good sources of EFAs.**

Secondly, fat is needed to absorb the fat-soluble vitamins from the food you eat. Without the fat, the vitamins go out the natural way. Without fat, absorbing fat-soluble vitamins is like trying to fetch water without a bucket. Last but not least, fat is what adds most of the flavor to your food. Without fat, most of what you eat would be pretty bland and boring.

Fat is good for you, as long as you don't take it overboard. Any less and you're most likely not getting enough. Any more, and you run the risk of packing on the love handles. And of the fat you DO eat, always strive to keep as much of it to be from the poly- and unsaturated fats. Don't go nuts about having a yolk or some peanut-butter once in a while, it's perfectly Ok as long as you don't lose sight of the big picture.

Reducing fat in your diet

By now you know that too much fat—especially saturated fat—is not good for you. Your body can easily store excess calories from fat as body fat. Plus, saturated fats from animal products, such as meats and dairy foods, can clog your arteries and contribute to heart disease.

But be careful. Although reducing dietary fat is important, eliminating all fat from your diet is not at all healthy. Fat is an essential nutrient that produces energy for daily activities and supplies the body with vitamins A, D and E, which are needed for healthy skin and optimal growth. The body cannot produce fat on its own; it must be provided through dietary intake. For these reasons you should enjoy some fats in your diet, especially monounsaturated fats like olive oil. The key is moderation—not elimination.

Research indicates that an excessive intake of saturated fats tends to raise blood cholesterol levels, thereby increasing risk for heart disease. Animal products—such as beef, butter, dairy products and lard—typically contain more saturated fat than do vegetable products. But some vegetable oils, such as coconut and palm oil (also known as tropical oils), contain large amounts of saturated fat.

There's also an unclassified newcomer in the fat realm—trans fatty acid. Trans fatty acids are the end products of a process called hydrogenation, in which vegetable oils are hardened. The implications that trans fatty acids may play a negative role on health is currently being reviewed, but many nutrition professionals are already advising a limited intake.

Health authorities recommend that Americans consume 20 percent or less of their total daily calories from fat, with 10 percent or less of those calories from saturated fat. Use the Nutrition Facts panel on food labels to help determine how much fat is in food. The following chart can help guide your fat intake. Determine how many calories are in your diet and use the chart to discover how many grams of fat are in 20 percent and 10 percent of your calorie intake. Remember, the recommended percentages refer to your total fat intake over time, not the fat in single foods or meals.

Calories per Day	Total Fat per Day (grams)	Total Saturated Fat per Day (grams)
1,200	26 or less	13 or less
1,600	36 or less	18 or less
2,000	44 or less	22 or less
2,200	48 or less	24 or less
2,500	54 or less	27 or less

10 tips to reduce fat

To help cut down on your fat intake, use the following tips when preparing foods:

1. Use evaporated skim milk instead of cream when preparing sauces or desserts.

2. Create your own nonfat salad dressing by mixing balsamic vinegar, mustard and herbs. If you really prefer an oil-based dressing, try using three parts vinegar to one part oil.

3. Drain nonfat yogurt through a sieve or cheesecloth overnight in the refrigerator, and use in recipes that call for cream.

4. Saute foods in chicken broth, vegetable stock, tomato juice or wine instead of frying them in oil or butter.

5. Keep olive oil in a spray bottle to a lightly coat sauté pans.

6. You can make your own taco shells. Hang soft corn tortillas directly over the oven rack (with the sides of the tortilla hanging down) and bake at 400 degrees until they're crisp. (Taco shells sold in supermarkets are usually fried.)

7. Whip up your own French fries. Place 1/4-inch-thick potato slices on a nonstick baking pan and coat with a light spray of oil. Sprinkle with paprika or salt, and bake at 350 degrees for 35 to 40 minutes. Turn once during baking.

8. To maximize flavor, toast nuts before baking with them. That way, you'll be able to use less. Or sprinkle nuts on top of a home-baked dessert instead of mixing them into the batter.

9. Substitute six egg whites plus one whole egg for every three eggs in your favorite recipes.

10. Substitute an equal amount of applesauce or any baby-food fruits for up to half of the total oil in your favorite dessert recipes. Strained prunes actually enhance the chocolate flavor in brownies!

Why eating excess fat makes us fat

While most of us know that consuming excessive amounts of fat will make us fat, we don't all understand exactly why this is true. To implement a successful weight management program, you need a good understanding of fat and why this nutrient makes us fat.

The amount of energy a particular food has depends on the quantity of fat, carbohydrates, and protein it contains. Food energy, both in its consumption and expenditure, is measured in terms of calories. Foods are either made up of fats, protein, carbohydrates, or a combination. A food that contains mostly fat will contain more than twice the calories than a food containing mostly carbohydrates and/or protein. For example, compare a serving of low-fat yogurt to a serving of nonfat yogurt—the low-fat yogurt has quite a few more calories than the nonfat variety because every gram of fat has more than twice the calories of a gram of protein or carbohydrate.

No more than 20 percent of your total calories should come from fat, fewer than 10 percent from saturated fat, the most damaging form. A recent study of 23 lean men and 23 obese men found little difference in the total number of calories each group consumed. But the obese men consumed, on average, more than 33 percent of their total calories from fat, compared with 19 percent for the lean men. Because the body converts dietary fat into body fat more easily than it converts protein and carbohydrates into body fat, the obese men were storing more fat even though both groups consumed the same total number of calories.

During the process of converting protein and carbohydrates to fat, your body uses them as energy and burns more than a quarter of their calories; it takes more energy (calories "burned") to convert carbohydrates and protein into body fat than it does to convert dietary fat into body fat. Thus, more carbohydrate and protein calories are used and fewer are stored as fat. Dietary fat, on the other hand, goes straight into storage, with very few calories being used. For example, Joe consumes 2,000 calories a day of which 40 percent come from fat. If Joe replaces half of the fat calories (20 percent of total calories) with calories coming from complex carbohydrates, less food will be converted to body fat even though the total number of calories consumed has not changed.

It is important to note that when that 20 percent of the 2,000 calories from fat now comes from carbohydrates (or protein), you consume a lot more food, since each gram of carbohydrate or protein contains less than half as many calories per gram. Therefore, when you begin to decrease the amount of fat in your diet and replace it with carbohydrates and protein, even if you still consume the same amount of food as before, you will be consuming a lot fewer calories.

If dietary fat were easy to control, most "diets" would probably succeed. Even with the recent explosion of low-fat and nonfat products, people generally still eat too much fat. The reason is simple: We have grown up loving fat, and we are accustomed to its taste and texture. Although most people do not usually crave fat as they do sugar or salty foods, we do have a strong taste preference for fat. Fat is responsible for the flavor and texture of many of our favorite foods: meats, cheese, dressings, sauces, creams, desserts, etc.

Because a high-fat diet increases fat storage and yields more than twice the amount of calories, the most effective way to reduce body fat is to concentrate on reducing your daily fat intake. Even if you do not consciously lower your total caloric intake, making the switch to a low-fat diet will most likely result in fat loss. However, attempts to suddenly restrict high-fat foods when you still have a strong preference for them causes feelings of deprivation which may, in turn, cause a higher intake of fat than normal.

Deprivation is part of the "diet" process, and one of the main reasons it is doomed to fail. It is very important to make gradual, healthier changes to the foods you enjoy.

Drastic changes backfire. When people base their food choices on the number of calories consumed and a "foods allowed/not allowed" list, the focus is on numbers rather than satiety and enjoyment of the foods' taste and texture. This often negates any positive effect the original focus on choosing low-fat foods may have had. Simply counting calories and grams of fat does not make for a permanent healthy lifestyle change. If tastes do not shift to enjoying foods lower in fat, this quickly becomes too restrictive and normal eating habits resume.

I'm not saying that you should avoid counting grams of fat altogether. The way to lower fat in your diet is to become a fat-conscious eater—and this requires that you know the amount of fat in each food. However, instead of counting fat grams and deciding if it is a "good food" or a "bad food," try to balance the foods you are eating so that you average 20 percent or less of your total calories from fat each day. It's okay to have a piece or two of high-fat pizza if you are truly hungry and craving it, as long as you balance that out with low-fat foods at other meals soon after. What's crucial is to learn how to make small healthier changes. Consume fat in moderation by balancing higher fat foods with lower fat foods.

You should now have a better understanding of fat and why excess consumption of this nutrient makes us fat. Your greatest challenge, however, is not learning new low-fat shopping or cooking techniques. Nor is it remembering how to calculate fat percentages or what to say to the waiter to reduce the fat in your restaurant meal. The greatest challenge facing you at this moment is deciding whether you are willing to make a change—to make small, gradual changes to the foods you love.

Sure, there is plenty of work to be done, but it really doesn't matter how long this new process takes. If you allow changes to take place over several years, your body will adjust comfortably, and you will be more likely to maintain the healthy lifestyle permanently. When you begin achieving improvements in energy and physical and psychological performance, the fun and excitement you experience will make the change well worth the effort. Action creates motivation!

What is the best ratio of macronutrtients?

Let start off by saying there is no "right" answer. The experts in the health and fitness community often debate the recommended ratio, of protein, carbohydrates, and fat to effectively build muscle and lose body fat. The amount you need is based on your own body's ability to metabolize nutrients and on your particular fitness goals. Again, experimentation is needed on your part here.

Don't get overwhelmed by trying to nail down an exact percentage! In the big picture, over the course of time a 10 percent difference or swing in a couple of the macronutrients is really not a big deal; especially if it causes you to procrastinate from starting your diet! If you are truly committed, you will have plenty of time to make adjustments when you pay close attention to your body.

This is how I keep it simple in my mind: As a bodybuilder, I must eat more protein than an average person. My secondary focus is consuming enough carbohydrates to have enough energy to train hard, prevent the body from ever using muscle as an energy source, and fuel my regular lifestyle activities. I sometimes add fat to my diet for energy or eliminate it altogether depending on how lean I want to be at the time.

From that basic rationale, you can see that I don't necessarily worry about an exact ratio of macronutrients to gain quality muscle mass and reduce body fat. **The percentages, however, normally end up being around 50 percent protein, 35 percent carbohydrates, and 15 percent fat.**

Meals; how many per day should I eat?

After you've estimated the total amount of calories that you need to eat each day, decided on the right ratio of protein, carbohydrates, and fat, you need to commit to an eating schedule, which spreads that food evenly throughout the day.

How many meals should you eat? That will depend on your time constraints and the total daily calories you allow yourself to eat. **A good rule of thumb would be to eat smaller, more frequent meals.** A dedicated bodybuilder should eat *at least* five times a day and space those meals no further than three hours apart.

> Doctor's Prescription:
> Depending on your schedule, make sure you eat 5-7 meals per day. Spread out your protein consumption evenly over the meals so you can keep a constant flow of amino acids in your system.

I eat 7 meals a day that are spread out every 2.5 hours. I've been eating this way for years. It's difficult at times because eating so frequently interrupts my train of thought and activities. But, because I am committed to becoming the best drug-free bodybuilder that I can be, that's a price I'm willing to pay.

The theory behind this way of eating is this: I have found eating smaller, more frequent meals, or in other words **"grazing" throughout the day, is the most efficient way for my body to process food.** Even though I may eat 7 meals a day, my total amount of calories of those meals only adds up to around 2,700 - 3,200 calories. 7 meals, totaling 3,000 calories, are far more efficient for the body to handle than only three meals totaling 3,000 calories.

Calculate the amount of protein, carbs, and fat in food

Before calculating the percentages of each of the macronutrients (protein, carbohydrates, and fat) make up of your total food intake, you must know the calorie conversion of each of them. A calorie is a unit to state the heat content of food. In simple terms, it is the amount of energy needed to "burn up" that type of food and amount of food.

Calorie Conversion

One calorie of protein is equal to 4 grams.
One calorie of carbohydrate is equal to 4 grams.
One calorie of fat is equal to 9 grams.

If you want 50 percent of the 2,500 calories you've allowed yourself for the day to come from protein, simply multiply 2,500 by 0.5. That means 1,250 of your 2,500 calories would come from protein. If you divide those 1,250 calories by 4 (the amount of grams one calorie of protein is equal to), you'll determine that you need 312.5 grams of protein every day. If you eat 7 meals a day and feel you should distribute protein evenly throughout the day, each of those 7 meals would consist of about 45 grams.

If you want 35 percent of the 2,500 calories you've allowed yourself for the day to come from carbohydrates, multiply 2,500 by 0.35. Which means 875 of your 2,500 calories would come from carbohydrates. If you divide those 875 calories by 4 (the amount of grams one calorie of carbohydrate is equal to), you'll determine that you need 218.75 grams of carbohydrates every day. If you eat 7 meals a day and feel you should distribute your carbohydrates evenly throughout the day, each of those 7 meals would consist of about 31 grams.

If you want 15 percent of the 2,500 calories you've allowed yourself for the day to come from fat, multiply 2,500 by 0.15. Which means 375 of your 2,500 calories would come from fat. If you divide those 375 calories by 9 (the amount of grams one calorie of fat is equal to), you'll determine that you need about 42 grams of fat every day. If you eat 7 meals a day and feel you should distribute your fat evenly throughout the day, each of those 7 meals would consist of about 5 grams.

Notice the totals of 45 grams of protein, 31 grams of carbohydrates, and 5 grams of fat that we determined each meal will consist of are very close to the nutritional breakdown of a typical meal replacement shake.

You can check your work by adding the amount of calories you have determined for each of the macronutrients are equal to the daily total of calories for the day in this manner:

Total protein (50%): 1,250
Total carbohydrates (35%): 875
Total fat (15%): 375

Total calories for the day: 2,500

Determining your maintenance level

For clarification purposes, your *maintenance* level is the amount of calories you need to stay at your *current* body weight. If you want to gain weight or lose weight, you'll obviously need to make adjustments.

There's really no way of determining *exactly* how many calories you should eat to maintain your current body weight, but here is a method that can get you close to your maintenance level. This method of calculation is called the *Harris-Benedict Equation.* This formula takes into account your sex, age, height, and weight. Other factors are considered as well.

Your heart, breathing, and mental activity all require energy (or calories). Even when you are resting, your body is burning calories to maintain its basic functions. This additional energy requirement is also taken into account by the *Harris-Benedict Equation.*

For men, the equation works as follows: First, multiply your weight by 13.8. Secondly, multiply your height (in inches) by 5. Next, multiply your age by 6.8 then subtract that figure from 67. Add these three totals together.

Here is an example of a 180 pound, 5'9", 23 year-old man:

180 pounds x 13.8 = 2,484.0
69 inches (5'9") x 5 = 345.0
23 years-old x 6.8 = 156.40
67 - 156.4 = - 89.4
____

Total Calories Needed: 2,739.6

For women, the equation works as follows: First, multiply your weight by 9.6. Secondly, multiply your height (in inches) by 1.8. Next, multiply your age by 4.7 then subtract that figure from 65.5. Add these three totals together.

Here is an example of a 120 pound, 5'3", 26 year-old woman:

120 pounds x 9.6 = 1,152.0
63 inches (5'3") x 1.8 = 113.4
26 years-old x 4.7 = 122.2
655 - 122.2 = 532.8
____

Total Calories Needed: 1,798.2

Of course, **this method can only *estimate*** the amount of calories you need to maintain your current weight. You may need to make some adjustments depending on the amount of exercise you do, the type of exercise, and your own individual metabolic factors.

Another way to determine your maintenance level

As I stated earlier, there's really no way of determining *exactly* how many calories you should eat to maintain your current body weight. Here's the challenge. Caloric requirements can change from person to person. Caloric requirements can also change from time period to time period within the same person. You may need to make some adjustments depending on the amount of exercise you do, the type of exercise, and your own individual metabolic factors.

I have a method to make the process of determining the amount of calories you should eat much simpler and probably just as effective.

1. Get a book with a complete listing of foods, their calories, and macronutrient breakdown.

2. Using the information I've provided in the previous section, decide on an appropriate breakdown of macronutrients for your daily food intake. Don't worry about being exact; you can make changes later if necessary.

3. Decide on the number of meals you are committed to eating each day.

4. This may sound too simple, but just pick a total number of calories you'll eat each day and divide that number by the number of meals you are committed to eating. This will give you the total number of calories you should plan to eat during each meal. After determining the amount of calories you should eat each meal, get your complete book of foods and plan your meals from there. 1500, 2000, 3000—whichever number you choose, you'll soon be able to figure out what adjustments you need to make.

<u>Importance of post workout nutrition</u>

<u>Invest your time wisely</u>

You don't need to be a resource management specialist to know that time is the most valuable finite resource that you have. And as you well know, there's a very limited amount of it to go around. So if you're smart, you'll figure out ways to get the greatest return on the investment of your time.

While this may be well recognized and applied in many aspects of modern life, it confuses me as to why people seem to ignore this when it comes to their exercise training. From what I see on a daily basis, it's clear to me that most people in the gym are wasting their time investment. They're spending precious hours engaged in strength or endurance training programs that yield little or no results?

Need proof? When was the last time someone in your gym made any noticeable physical progress? In fact, when was the last time that you made any significant physical progress? Exercise training has the potential to yield huge returns on any given time investment. Isn't it a shame that most people don't ever see this magnitude of return?

* * *

The Doctor Says:

I know I sound like a motivational speaker or a financial planner when I say this but you do need to use your time to your advantage. The proper use of your time is the single biggest factor whether you will be a success or failure in life.

* * *

Despite this disappointing reality, I'm here to tell you that hope is not lost. In fact, there's a very easy way to capitalize on your investment. You see, in most cases the exercise is not the problem. The problem is that people fail to invest in the other important commodity that, in combination with exercise, yields the biggest returns.

They're buying the cart without the horse, the lemonade stand without the lemonade. They're spending their time focused on only the exercise program while ignoring the importance of a sound nutritional program.

Now I could write a dozen articles focused on straightening out the nutritional problems of the world. But those articles are for another day. Today I intend to focus on what is, in my opinion, the most important aspect of exercise nutrition; eating during the post-workout period. The knowledge of how to eat during this time will maximize your efforts in the gym and yield the biggest returns on your time investment.

Remodeling the post-workout period

Exercise, both strength and endurance training, are responsible for countless health and aesthetic benefits. However the exercise itself is a significant physiological stressor.

Perceived symptoms of this "stress" are often mild and include muscle soreness, the need for extra sleep, and an increased appetite.

These symptoms let us know that the exercise has depleted the muscle's fuel resources, caused some minor damage, and that the muscle is in need of replenishment and repair. While the words depletion and damage may sound like negative things, they're not if they only stick around for a short period of time. You see, these changes allow the muscle to adapt by getting better at the exercise demands placed on it.

Therefore if you're doing endurance exercise, the muscle will become depleted and damaged in the short run, but in the long run it will super compensate, building itself up to be a better aerobic machine. And if strength training is your thing, you'll tear down you're weaker muscle fibers in favor of building up bigger, stronger ones.

In all cases, exercise essentially tears down old, less adapted muscle in order to rebuild more functional muscle. This phenomenon is called remodeling. While the remodeling process is much more complex than I can describe here, it's important for me to emphasize that this remodeling only takes place if the muscle is provided the right raw materials. If I plan on remodeling my home I can hire a guy to tear down a couple of walls, a guy to clean up the mess, and a guy to come in and rebuild better walls than the ones that came down. But if I don't give that guy any bricks, how's he going to get anything done? If I don't give him the bricks, all I'll have in the end is a much smaller, unfinished house.

The same holds true with exercise remodeling. In particular, during the exercise bout and the time immediately following it, exercise breaks down our muscle carbohydrate stores and our muscle protein structures. Then, the immune system comes in to clean up the mess. And finally, signals are generated to tell the body to rebuild. However, without the proper protein and carbohydrate raw materials, this building can't take place. You'll be left with muscles that never reach their potential.

So with this analogy, I hope it's obvious that this post-exercise period is not a time to take lightly. Remember, you spent a significant amount of time in the gym breaking down the muscle for a good reason. You want it to be better adapted to future demands. So to realize full return on your time investment, you need to give the body the raw materials it needs, namely protein and carbohydrates.

You have to feed your hungry muscles

As I mentioned, all trainees (male or female), regardless of their chosen mode of exercise, must take their post-exercise nutrition seriously in order to provide the muscle with the raw materials it needs. As all types of exercise use carbohydrates for energy, muscle carbohydrate depletion is inevitable. Therefore a post-workout meal high in carbohydrates is required to refill muscle carbohydrate/energy stores.

However any ol' amount of carbohydrates will not do. You need to consume enough carbohydrates to promote a substantial insulin release. **Insulin is the hormone responsible for shuttling carbohydrates and amino acids into the muscle.** In doing this, carbohydrate re-synthesis is accelerated and protein balance becomes positive, leading to rapid repair of the muscle tissue.

$$* * *$$

Doctor's Prescription:

After your workout is the best time for simple carbohydrates because your muscles are starving for energy. I recommend a Gatorade type of simple carb drink, even pop if it's the only thing available.

$$* * *$$

Therefore, **by consuming a large amount of carbohydrates, you will promote a large insulin release, increase glycogen storage, and increase protein repair.** Research has shown that a carbohydrate intake of 0.8 to 1.2 grams per 1 kilogram of body weight, for your post workout meal, maximizes glycogen synthesis and accelerates protein repair. However, unless you've had a very long, intense workout, 1.2g/kg may be a bit excessive as excess carbohydrate can be converted to body fat. Therefore I recommend 0.9g of carbohydrate per 1 kilogram of body weight for speeding up muscle carbohydrate replenishment while preventing excess fat gain.

In addition, since muscle protein is degraded during exercise, the addition of a relatively large amount of protein to your post exercise meal is necessary to help rebuild the structural aspects of the muscle. After exercise, the body decreases its rate of protein synthesis and increases its rate of protein breakdown. However, the provision of protein and amino acid solutions has been shown to reverse this trend, increasing protein synthesis and decreasing protein breakdown.

$$* * *$$

Doctor's Prescription:

Along with the simple carbs post-workout, you need a heavy dose of protein at this time too. Protein, especially after an exhausting workout, has a muscle sparing effect (saves your muscles from being broken down in to amino acids).

$$* * *$$

Researchers have used anywhere from 0.2g - 0.4g of protein per 1 kilogram of body weight to demonstrate the effectiveness of adding protein to a post-workout carbohydrate drink. As an increased consumption of the essential amino acids may lead to a more positive protein balance, 0.4g/kg may be better than 0.2g/kg.

While your post-workout feeding should be rich protein and carbohydrate, this meal should be fat free. The consumption of essential fats is one of the most overlooked areas of daily nutritional intake but during the post workout period, eating fat can actually decrease the effectiveness of your post-workout beverage. Since fat slows down transit through the stomach, eating fat during the post workout period may slow the digestion and absorption of carbohydrates and proteins. As your post workout feeding should be designed to promote the most rapid delivery of carbohydrates and protein to your depleted muscles, fats should be avoided during this time.

Finally, another important factor to consider is the timing of this meal. **It is absolutely crucial that you consume your post-workout meal immediately after exercise.** As indicated above, after exercise, the muscles are depleted and require an abundance of protein and carbohydrate. In addition, during this time, the muscles are biochemically "primed" for nutrient uptake.

This phenomenon is commonly known as the "window of opportunity". Over the course of the recovery period, this window gradually closes and by failing to eat immediately after exercise, you diminish your chances of promoting full recovery. To illustrate how quickly this window closes, research has shown that **consuming a post-exercise meal immediately after working out is superior to consuming one only 1 hour later.** In addition, consuming one 1 hour later is superior to consuming one 3 hours later. If you wait too long, glycogen replenishment and protein repair will be compromised.

So, when you decided to start exercising you decided to give up a specific amount of time per week in the interest of getting better, physically. However, if you haven't spent the necessary time thinking about post-exercise nutrition, you're missing much of the benefit that comes with exercising. I assure you that once you start paying attention to this variable in the recovery equation, your time in the gym will be much better invested. The results you will obtain will be all the proof you need.

Whole food vs. protein drinks

Anchored firmly atop their calorie-counting soapbox, nutritionists have traditionally asserted that whole food always trumps supplemental nutrition. For them I have only one sentiment: "Always…it is a meaningless word." -Oscar Wilde

While I wholeheartedly believe that complete, unbleached, untreated, and unprocessed whole food should form the basis of any sound nutritional regimen, there are some instances in which supplements can actually be superior to whole food. In the case of post-exercise nutrition, I believe that liquid supplemental nutrition is far superior to whole food for the following reasons.

* * *

Doctor's Prescription:

Use liquid meals (i.e. protein drinks) when it is beneficial to your body and your schedule to do so. Also, filling in some of the snacks in-between your whole food meals with protein drinks is a good way to keep your protein intake spread out.

* * *

Liquid meals taste good and are getting better

Typically, after intense exercise, most people complain that eating a big meal is difficult. This is understandable as the exercise stress creates a situation where the hunger centers are all but shut down. However, as you now know, it's absolutely critical that you eat if you want to remodel the muscle, enlarge the muscle, or recover from the exercise.

Fortunately liquid supplemental formulas are palatable, easy to consume, and can be quite nutrient dense, providing all the nutrition you need at this time. In addition, since these formulas are structurally simple; the gastrointestinal tract has no difficulty processing them. **Your stomach will thank you for this.**

Liquid meals have a fast absorption profile

The latest research has demonstrated that liquid supplemental formulas containing fast digesting protein (whey hydrolysates and isolates) and carbohydrates (dextrose and maltodextrin) are absorbed more quickly than whole food meals. To put this into perspective, **a liquid post-exercise formula may be fully absorbed within 30 to 60 minutes,** providing much needed muscle nourishment by this time. However, a slower digesting solid food meal may take 2 to 3 hours to fully reach the muscle.

Liquid meals take advantage of the window of opportunity

The faster the protein and carbohydrates get to the muscle, the better your chances for muscle building and recovery. Speed is of the essence when it comes to using your window of opportunity. Current research has demonstrated that subjects receiving nutrients within one hour after exercise recover more quickly than subjects receiving nutrients three hours after exercise. Liquid nutrition is making more sense, isn't it?

Liquid meals are better for nutrient targeting

During the post exercise period, specific nutrients maximize your recovery. These include an abundance of water, high glycemic index carbohydrates, and certain amino acids. It's also best to avoid fat during this time. So the only way to ensure that these nutrients are present in the right amounts is to formulate a specific liquid blend. Whole foods may miss the mark.

Main points for building muscle

High-intensity for bodybuilding involves the application of maximum effort to build maximum muscle in minimum time. High-intensity training bodybuilders don't waste energy trying out the latest super routines in the muscle magazines. They don't train "instinctively." They generally don't squander training times with pumping exercises. They don't adopt the attitude that performing a few extra sets will make up for earlier sets that were poorly executed.

Instead, successful high-intensity training bodybuilders focus mostly on compound exercises such as the dead lift, squat, bent over row, leg press, and other heavy movements. These bodybuilders endeavor to gradually build their poundages by adding a repetition or so each workout and/or increasing the weight by small increments as often as possible, because they know that **getting stronger on the big movements is the best way to stimulate real gains in size.** They know exactly what exercises and weights they are going to use when they arrive at the gym. They strive to get the most out of every repetition and every set.

High-intensity training bodybuilding comprises the soundest application of the principles of exercise physiology. It's a methodical, disciplined, uncomplicated approach to physique development. If you are a drug-free trainee interested in maximizing your natural bodybuilding potential, **high-intensity training is the fastest route to your destination.**

Keep volume low and intensity high

Some claim that you must do a certain number of sets per body part to induce muscular growth. While it's true that the volume of work performed is a consideration, if volume were the primary stimulus for growth then marathon runners would have massively muscle legs. Instead, a casual observation of distance runners almost always reveals thin legs that appear nearly devoid of appreciable muscle.

Intensity that is, the amount of effort applied to each set, supersedes volume when it comes to producing results. Coupled with the gradual progression in poundage, intensity is the key to growth. In fact, one set performed at 100 percent intensity is far more productive than 10 sets performed at 75 percent intensity.

100 percent intensity means performing a set until you are unable, despite your most aggressive effort, to squeeze out one more repetition with good form. This is also known as training to muscle fatigue or failure. It is simple in concept but difficult in execution. Most trainees who think that they are training to fatigue actually terminate their sets well before reaching true fatigue, particularly when it comes to heavy leg exercises. The mind gives out before the body.

High-intensity training bodybuilding is based upon the notion that muscular growth is the result of the body's effort to protect itself from the stress of training heavy. **The more intense the stress, the greater the body's protective response.** This is why the highest possible intensity, taking each work set to the point of muscular fatigue, is required for the fastest progress.

Pushing each set to muscular failure is the most efficient way to train because it ensures the greatest numbers of muscle fibers are stimulated within the shortest amount of time and with the lowest possible volume of work. The all-or-none principle of muscle fiber recruitment states that a muscle uses only the minimum number of fibers necessary to complete a given task and that those fibers contract with maximal force. As you proceed through a set, the muscle fibers that initially lifted the weight become fatigued, forcing fresh fibers to assist in continuing the set. By the time you reach muscular fatigue, most or all of the target muscle fibers have been exhausted. Training to fatigue also ensures that you use the heaviest possible weight for the given number of repetitions. Both of these scenarios set the stage for the fastest possible growth.

This begs the question: if one set to fatigue is good, aren't two sets better and 10 sets better still? No. Performing an excessive number of sets of the given exercise will not increase intensity, it increases volume. It's essential to understand that the body possesses a limited ability to cope with the demands of any stressor, including exercise. **The right amount of high-intensity training leads to results; too much high-intensity training leads to overtraining.** Needless to say, muscular growth will not occur in an overtrained body.

Train briefly and infrequently

Once you understand that training as hard as possible ensures maximum growth stimulation, the next point to grasp is that training as briefly as possible ensures the body has the resources it needs to provide growth. Bear in mind that the body's first priority after a workout is to recover the energy expended during that workout. Only after the body returns to its pre-workout state will it begin the process of supercompensation or growth. It stands to reason that trainees should **perform the minimum amount of work required to stimulate growth to preserve enough energy to foster the growth process.**

There exists no ideal workout length or set. These parameters vary among trainees, depending upon the individual genetic makeup, training history, and lifestyle. But it's safe to say that if you're training in proper high-intensity training style, one or two sets of any exercise is plenty, with six sets being the maximum one should perform for any single body part. Less is probably better for most people.

In general, two workouts per week or a workout every three to four days is sufficient for most to make progress. This applies to advanced trainees as well as beginners. In fact, advanced trainees may need to workout even less often than beginners because their increased strength and ability to generate more effort places their bodies under greater stress. Whatever frequency you initially choose, you should **add more rest days between your workouts if you find that you're still tired and sore by the time of your next workout** or if you fail to increase poundages/repetitions regularly.

Train for strength

Imagine that you currently bench press a maximum of 250 pounds for eight repetitions. You spend the next 12 months performing continuous tension, muscle confusion, and other alleged muscle building techniques. At the end of the twelve-month period, you can still bench press a maximum of 250 pounds for eight repetitions. How much muscle to think you'll have gained? The answer is none. Yes, none, even after years' worth of effort.

That's because a relationship exists between the muscle strength and its size. Sadly, many trainees never comprehend this reality. Instead of making a conscious effort to increase their poundages regularly, they fall into the trap of trying every new technique glorified in the bodybuilding magazines. But because they don't get stronger, they don't get bigger.

Don't be swayed by the throng of so-called bodybuilders who perform set after set of an exercise with the goal of achieving a maximum pump. **A pump has nothing to do with true growth; it is merely a temporary state in which the muscle is engorged with blood.**

If you want to build real, lasting muscle tissue, you must make the muscle stronger. This means training for strength. When you're able to do the target number of repetitions with the given weight, it's time to increase that weight. This increase should be small, about five to ten pounds for leg exercises and 2 1/2 to five pounds on upper body exercises is usually enough.

Most people, when they even bother to increase their weights, make the mistake of increasing them too much. This leads to a rapid deterioration of form. Don't be impatient; overtime, small increases add up to a large increase.

Use an appropriate repetition range

Many authorities believe that hypertrophy can be maximized by repetitions in the range of about 8 to 12. This is a useful principle to follow but, in truth, there can be a significant difference in productive repetition ranges among individuals and among body parts within the same individual.

In general, sets of about five repetitions or less should be avoided by bodybuilders because such low repetitions demonstrate strength rather than build it. In addition, sets of about five repetitions or less at a typical cadence heavily stress the joints and connective tissue without keeping the muscle fibers loaded long enough to provoke growth. Sets of about 15 repetitions or more promote greater metabolic and muscular endurance adaptations rather than strength/growth. **This leaves a usable repetition range for bodybuilding purposes of about 6 to 15.**

A compelling amount of evidence suggests that the lower body responds better than the upper body to higher repetition ranges. As such, it may be best use about 10 to 15 repetitions for lower body work and about 6 to 10 repetitions for upper body work. Experiment with both the upper and lower end of these repetition ranges to discover what works best for you.

Focus on the major muscle groups

If you want to get bigger, you are going to have to pay the price in the form of agonizing effort on exercises that allow you to use relatively heavy weights. The focus should be on compound movements that works several muscle groups at the same time, such as the squat, deadlifts, chin up, bent over row, and bench press. In fact, a very productive routine that stimulates serious growth from head to toe can be built around just these five exercises.

That's not to say that calf raises, arm exercises, and abdominal work should be avoided. They can be part of your program, especially once you're an advanced trainee. Just understand that you'll simulate more biceps growth by doing heavy chin-ups and rows than you will by doing set after set of concentration curls.

The majority of the muscle mass on your body is found in your hips, legs, back, and chest. The only way to gain the pounds of muscular body weight that will accentuate your appearance is by increasing the size of these muscles. **Train the large muscle groups heavy and hard and the smaller groups will gain as well.**

Use proper training style and technique

For best results, it's not enough to lift heavy weights, you must lift them properly. Heaving, thrusting, jerking, and bouncing should be avoided at all costs. As a bodybuilder, your mission in the gym is to exhaust your muscles so that they are forced to rebuild larger and stronger. Weights and machines are the tools you used for that purpose. While you want to lift as much weight as possible for given number of repetitions, you want to do so within the context of proper form.

Jerky and bouncing motions may allow you to lift more weight than you otherwise might be able to handle but such motions minimize the load on the muscles you are trying to work. **Such motions also multiply the stress on your joints and connective tissue, setting you up for injury.**

Some training authorities suggest following a 2 to 4 protocol in which the positive motion takes two seconds in the negative motion takes four seconds. This is fine general advice but what's important to remember is that you want to keep the muscle loaded throughout the entire repetition. Lift the weight with power, precision, and focus; pause for second in the fully contracted position; and lower the weight reasonably slowly while feeling the muscle resist the weight all the way down.

Emphasize recovery more than you think you should

Training provides the stimulus for growth but the growth process does not take place while you train. It takes place later when you rest and especially when you sleep.

Taking an adequate number of days off between workouts is only part of the recovery equation. You must also ensure that your rest days are truly rest days. **If your goal is to add substantial muscle to your frame, minimize your activity level outside the gym.** Playing full-court basketball may be fun but doing so regularly will deplete energy that would otherwise be directed toward recovery and supercompensation. Determine your priorities and act accordingly.

Nor can you afford to frolic until the wee hours of the morning if your dream is to get big. Sleep is critical to the growth process and must not be overlooked. Six hours a night is the bare minimum you should sleep and seven or eight hours is preferable. **Understand that even the most painstakingly devised and religiously followed training program will yield little or no gains if you're sleep deprived.**

Eat well and often

If training serves as the catalyst for growth and sleep provides the opportunity for growth, and food provides the raw materials required for growth.

The ideal eating plan to get big is based around lean protein sources (lean beef, chicken breast, turkey breast, fish, egg whites, and low-fat dairy products), complex carbohydrates (oatmeal, brown rice, yams, and potatoes), fibrous carbohydrates (vegetables and whole fruits), and a small to moderate amount of healthy fats (egg yolks, vegetable oils, nuts, and nut butters). The occasional addition, perhaps a few times weekly, of sweets and fast foods is fine, but keep in mind that a steady intake of sugar and fat laden foods can lead to a rapid accumulation of body fat.

Structure your eating plan to provide five to seven moderate size meals each day. **Smaller, more frequent feedings provide your muscles with a constant supply of the nutrients** they need for growth without promoting excessive fat storage. Such an eating plan will keep your energy level stable and minimize cravings.

Supplements such as protein powers and meal replacements should be viewed as conveniences rather than necessities. Natural food should form the cornerstones of your nutrition program, but when time is short a meal replacement or protein drink is preferable to fast food or no food.

Combine machines and free weights

The arguments in supporting both free weights and machines are loud and long. Free weight supporters claim that the balance required to lift free weights provide a stronger growth stimulus to the muscles and machine lovers point out that machine users can work their muscles harder precisely because they don't have to balance the weight. Free weights are said to be a more natural form of resistance while machines are designed to make up for the inherent shortcomings of barbells and dumbbells.

Each side as valid arguments, so why not get the benefits of both by combining free weights and machines in your program? A very productive routine can be designed around barbells, dumbbells, and whatever machines you have access to.

Keep a daily workout record

Most trainees have no idea where they're going to reach their destination because they don't keep track of where they've been. That is, they don't keep a training diary.

To make the most out of high-intensity bodybuilding, you're going to have to keep records. Don't trust your memory; put your performances on paper. For every work set completed, you should write down the weights used and repetitions obtained. Refer to your training diary during your next training session and try as hard as possible to better your previous performance.

This implies, of course, that the only frequent changes in your routine should be in repetitions and poundages, not exercises. While some variety is reasonable, continually changing exercises doesn't give you the benefit of establishing linear progression from workout to workout, which is the basis for long-term improvement. This does not mean you should use the same exercises for years on end. It only means that you should stick with a given exercise until it ceases to work for you. Leave the so-called instinctive training principle, which states that one should "confuse" the muscles by constantly changing exercises from workout to workout, for those who are more interested in being a Poser than in making progress.

Diet to obtain muscular definition and low bodyfat

While getting bigger is the primary goal of the typical trainee, most serious bodybuilders eventually develop the urge to improve their muscular definition. After all, the source of the unique appearance of bodybuilders, the thing that distinguishes them from just another big person who pumps iron is crisp, sharply delineated musculature.

In truth, training for definition is a fallacy. **Definition is not a quality that can be trained into a muscle; it is nothing more than the absence of fat over a well-developed muscle.** The peaks, valleys, separations, and veins that characterize a detailed physique exist in anyone who has developed a respectable degree of muscle mass. If these muscular details cannot be seen, it's because they are obscured by bodyfat.

The best way to train for definition is to adopt a sensible fat loss plan. Put simply, you'll have to eat less. But you want to eat only a little less, starvation diets burn more muscle than fat. A slight reduction, perhaps 300 to 400 calories daily, should be sufficient to set the fat loss machinery in motion. Aim for a loss of just one pound weekly; more rapid weight loss will quickly eat into your hard earned muscle mass.

The best fat loss diets are based around frequent feedings. Eat five to seven small meals a day consisting of lean protein, a moderate amount of carbohydrates, and a small model fat. While mainstream nutritionists typically promote high carbohydrate eating plans, many competitive bodybuilders find that they get their best fat loss results by consuming a moderate amount of carbohydrates, perhaps 40 percent or less of their calories. These bodybuilders also find a better to taper their carbohydrates as the day goes on by eating starchy carbohydrates for breakfast and lunch and fibrous carbohydrates such as broccoli, a staple source of carbohydrates for bodybuilders, during the late afternoon in the evening.

A moderate amount of cardiovascular activity can assist in fat loss. Whether you choose to run or walk at a fast pace outdoors or indoors on a treadmill, or bike indoors or outdoors, or use one of the numerous cardio machines available at commercial gyms. **Start out by performing the activity two or three times weekly for 20 minutes at a moderate intensity.** Gradually increase the duration and number of cardio sessions. Since excessive cardiovascular work can cut into muscle size, perform the minimum amount of cardio activity required to keep fat loss occurring until you reach her goal. Try not to exceed five 45-minute cardio sessions weekly.

While trying to get lean, your approach to weight training should be the same as when you're striving to add mass: train intensely, briefly, and infrequently. At this point, increasing your volume is an even bigger mistake than it was when you training for size, as a decrease in caloric intake and the inclusion of cardio work makes you more susceptible to overtraining.

What about developing an impressive "six-pack" abdominal region? This again is a matter of eliminating excess body fat through diet and cardio. Performing countless crunches, setups, and leg raises in hopes of bringing out the abs is a waste of time and effort. As your percentage of body fat lowers, your abs will become more prominent. **To display a truly impressive rock hard mid-section, you'll need to lower your percentage of body fat too well under 10 percent**, and undertaking that requires discipline and diligence. **Women would need to drop their percentage of body fat to the low teens.**

I get bombarded with e-mails from all over the world, from Japan to Argentina, and it's interesting to see how small differences there are, really. Everybody wants to know how to get stronger and more buff. Everybody wants to lose body fat. Everybody wants to know if protein drinks really work. The last question is a simple "yes," but the two before that are little bit trickier.

Still, there are some more specific questions that inevitably pop up from time to time. Here are a few of them.

Q: My friend has really peaked biceps while mine are not, while we both curl the same weight. How come? What can I do to increase my peak?

A: Unfortunately, the shape of muscle is largely determined by genetics, so blame mom and dad. However, there are some things you can do. The biceps consists of two separate heads, and by smart training you can develop both to their limit. Don't expect to be able to solely pinpoint one of the two, but you can shift the focus a little. One exercise I have found particularly well for bringing out the peak is bicep curls with a straight barbell, where you hold the bar with a more-than-shoulder-width grip and tuck in your elbows against your sides. Experiment a little to see what works best for you. Start with slightly less weight than usual and do 12-15 reps just to feel where the burn materializes. Then flex your biceps in a classic bicep-pose and use your other hand to squeeze the peak of your biceps. If that's where the lactic acid burn is at, you've found an exercise that will work.

Q: I have a horrible sweet tooth, but I need to get in shape. What can I do to avoid going crazy?

A: Use the window of opportunity immediately after your workouts to have a handful or two of candy. As I've talked about before, that is the one time when you should be eating something sugary to get your body back into an anabolic state again. Make sure to get something sugary though, not fat. Fat has a lot more calories per gram than sugar, and fat will slow down the release of the sugars into your blood stream. Examples of good candy: Jelly beans, sugar babies and reduced fat cookies. Examples of bad candy: Chocolate, candy bars and peanut-butter cups.

Q: You say I should do lat pull-downs to the front rather than behind the neck. Why?

A: To work the lats effectively, you must keep your back slightly arched. By pulling the bar to the front, you're all but guaranteed to keep the arch, while a pull behind the neck lends itself to cheating as you get tired. Thereby you could routinely rob yourself of the benefit from the last few reps of each set without even knowing it. In addition, it's a more natural movement to pull the bar to the front. Your shoulders are at less of a vulnerable angle, and as you get stronger you might avoid cumulative shoulder injuries. This is only true for some people, but the bad news is that you usually don't know if you're one of them until it's too late, so play it safe and assume that you are.

Last but not least, there is an important thing to notice about the lat pulls to the front. You might be tempted to lean back too much when you get tired, thus giving yourself an extra pull. Try to avoid this kind of swaying - sit upright with a lightly arched back, and stay that way throughout the exercise.

Q: What are your thoughts on sports drinks such as Gatorade, Hydra Fuel and such?

A: I don't have any problem with them as long as they're consumed in conjunction with hard and prolonged exercise. Most sports drinks are full of sugar and are formulated to replace lost fluid through sweating, so they're not suitable for drinking with your dinner. In the gym or on a field, they're perfectly fine. Just watch for artificial ingredients. If the drink has a long laundry-list of suspicious-sounding chemicals that you can't even pronounce, pick something else.

Q: My friend is considering buying some steroids, but is concerned about getting ripped off rather than getting the real thing. Is there any web site that can help you identify the legit labels and such?

A: Uh-huh. And I bet your "friend" is about your age and height too, right? Look, here's another reason not to take steroids: It's virtually impossible to know what you're taking. If the crook peddling this dope fills a vial with liquid cleaning agent and slaps a realistic-looking sticker on it, you wouldn't have a clue of what you injected until you woke up in the E.R. If you're lucky, that is. I've seen sites where they promise to show you the telltale signs of counterfeit labels, but guess what? The counterfeiters read the same advice! The bottom line is that all you have to go on is the word of the seller, and, quite frankly, do you think he cares more about your health than his own wallet? Really?

Q: I just can't seem to hit my rear delts properly, and that is getting more and more of a problem as my side and front delts grow. What can I do?

A: Try attaching a handle to the lower pulley on a pulley machine. Then kneel on the floor with your side turned to the pulley. Grab the handle with the hand furthest away from the pulley and lean forward so that you support your upper body with your free hand against the floor. Let the handle pull your other arm so that you feel a good stretch in the rear delt. In other words, if you got your right side facing the pulley, you hold the handle in your left hand while supporting yourself with the right hand on the floor. You should be so far away from the pulley machine that you have resistance even at your most stretched. Then simply pull the handle out to the side as far you can without moving or swaying the rest of your body. The only thing moving should be your shoulder and your arm. This way you can experiment with different angles and slight variations to hit the rear delts 100%.

Q: How important is warm-up, really? I know I'm supposed to do at least 5 minutes on the bike before I hit the weights, but I have very little time…

A: Let me put it this way: If you can "afford" 5 minutes more of watching TV, or 5 minutes of dozing after lunch, or whatever, you'd be better off spending those 5 minutes on a warm-up. Not only do you get your body going so that it utilizes fat for fuel better, it also drastically decreases your risk of injury - especially if you're planning on lifting big. There's no justification for skipping something that can do so much for your health and safety, unless you're a top-level executive who sleeps 3 hours per night and makes 15-minute appointments to play with your kids on the weekends. If you're a mere mortal like the rest of us, who spends a few hours in front of the tube now and then, you're making an active choice to watch TV instead of looking out for yourself. And by the way, don't you think a single torn muscle, with all the handicaps and rehab it involves, makes up for the time you'd save by skipping the warm-up during your entire life? Play it safe - always warm up.

Q: How come the people in before and after-pictures in the ads always look so much better than I do, no matter how hard I work out, diet, and take the supplements they push?

A: And drinking certain brands of soda doesn't make you an extreme-sporting mega hunk either, even if their ad implies so. Read the fine print. There's always a puny little disclaimer saying something to the effect of: "Mr. Ripped on the picture experienced exceptional results. The typical user may not expect similar results." In plain English, that means they all but admit that while the dude on a picture is a nice fairy tale, the Muscle Fairy will most likely visit not you. The sad truth is that there are no shortcuts. When an ad claims that their product is 3,463% better than the competition, it does not mean you'll gain muscle 3,463% faster. In fact, most scientific claims I've seen are taken out of context. Sure, a certain ingredient in product X may do a lot of good for an 80-year old female diabetic, or help an obese lab rat, but to expect even remotely the same results in a 230 lb, 25-year old male bodybuilder is ridiculous. Yet, they can quote the scientific study and advertise it to create the illusion that the 80-year old woman figures somehow applies to you. It's dirty, but it works. Otherwise they wouldn't keep doing it. Of course, there are honest facts in ads, and there are reputable companies who don't try to scam you with inflated claims, but it's generally easy to spot the difference. Remember: If something sounds too good to be true, it usually is.

Q: I have kind of an embarrassing problem… I don't use steroids, and still I've noticed my pecs are kind of "drooping" when relaxed, making them look like the beginning stages of breasts. I train religiously, I have very little body fat, and still I think it keeps getting worse! What's up with this??

A: Don't panic. What you're seeing is probably the effect of too much decline bench pressing. Lately, I've seen a surge the number of people using decline presses, the kind where you lock your legs between two rolls and lay with your head down on a declining bench. This often allows you to use slightly more weight in the bench press, which as we all know is the Holy Grail for 99% of the male gym rats ages 15 to 30. The bad news is; the pectoralis major has a fan-shape, allowing you to train different areas to different degrees. If you do a lot of incline presses, you're weaker compared to the flat press, but you train the upper part of your chest. This gives you a well-balanced, rock-solid look. However, if you train the lower part of your pecs too much, especially if neglecting the upper part, you grow the muscles into looking like a flat-chested dude with beginning bitch tits. Make sense? The muscles will grow according to how you train them, so my advice to you is to stop doing decline presses immediately, and focus on flat and incline presses for a couple of months. When you've balanced out and start feeling comfortable again, you can go back to a normal training routine again - splitting the focus equally between the upper and lower part of the chest.

Q: Why is breakfast so important?

A: When you've been asleep for 8 or so hours, you haven't eaten for at least 8 hours, possibly more like 10 or 11 hours. This means your body is really low on amino acids and carbs, both something you want to have floating around in your body to stay anabolic. The best way to break the starvation of your muscles is to have a hearty breakfast as soon as possible as you wake up. Also, if you work out early in the day, it's extra important to get a lot of carbs with your breakfast, as you'll need it to fuel your workout.

Q: What is the best repetition range for building muscle?

A: At an average repetition cadence (speed), generally 8 -12 reps per set will elicit the greatest gains in lean mass. Sets consisting of less than 6 or 8 reps generally focus on muscle strength, whereas a high number of reps each set targets muscle endurance.

Detailed Answer:

The conventional view that fewer reps in each set equates to more muscle gain is a bit too simplistic. In reality, when one performs sets with very high weight and low reps, the main physiological change is a strengthening of neuromuscular pathways. In other words, high weight/low reps strengthen the brain's ability to activate muscle. However, if we bump up the reps slightly while decreasing the weight as necessary, the muscle tissue will perform more total work, and thus more muscle growth will occur. However, if the reps are increased too high, the main effect will be an increase in muscle endurance.

Through research, it has been determined that the best range for hypertrophy (muscle gain) is roughly between 8-12 reps. As the reps are decreased from this range, the program will elicit greater strength gains will less size. In contrast, more than 12 reps mainly allows for increases in muscular endurance.

Q: Does weight training cause high blood pressure?

A: Natural bodybuilders are among the most fit individuals in athletics. While weight training itself has little effect on cardiovascular health, it does not increase blood pressure in the long term. Although blood pressure does rise during any type of exercise, which is not dangerous for healthy individuals. However, most bodybuilders also engage in cardiovascular exercise, which is well established for decreasing blood pressure.

Also, natural bodybuilders tend to be very lean; not only on the "outside," but also on the "inside," as they tend to have less fatty plaque lining artery walls, and are therefore at a reduced risk for atherosclerosis. Further, the "large heart syndrome" that many purport as a result of weight training has not been proven in research.

Q: Is it possible to gain muscle strength or muscle endurance without gaining muscle size?

A: It is possible to gain strength without increasing muscle size (hypertrophy). Similarly, it is possible to enhance muscle endurance without hypertrophy. However, it may be difficult to train for both goals at the same time.

- Training for muscle endurance is generally achieved through high repetitions and lighter weights.

- To train for strength while minimizing gains in muscle mass, it is advisable to perform low repetitions per set, using explosive movements (short concentric contractions) while lowering the weights under control. Be sure to be adequately warmed up before starting into the working sets.

Detailed Answer:

Training for strength over size is largely attained through manipulating the neuromuscular system (brain-muscle connection); that is, strengthening the nervous system as a muscle "activator". As a protective mechanism for the body, the central nervous system has safeguards in place that shut down muscle activity when the muscle attempts to work at too high an intensity.

Specifically, one of these systems works through an organelle found in tendons of muscle, which shuts down muscle activity when it senses that there is too much strain on a muscle. Also, for the untrained individual (or somebody who rarely lifts very heavy weights), the connection between muscle and brain may be relatively weak. To train the neuromuscular connection, it is advisable to perform low repetitions per set, using explosive movements (short concentric contractions) while lowering the weights under control.

Be sure to be adequately warmed up before starting into the working sets. Although muscle fiber density may increase from this type of training, hypertrophy is minimized since high resistance/low rep training does not elicit changes in extra-fibril structures (blood vessels, organelles like mitochondria). At the same time, strength gains will be evident through neuromuscular manipulation.

Training for muscle endurance is generally achieved through high repetitions and lighter weights. With this type of training, the major change to the muscle is the ability to manage metabolic waste, and fuel utilization. For example, the muscle is better able to utilize lactate as a fuel rather than allow it to minimize muscle performance.

Also, more efficient fuel sources such as fats make up a larger portion of the muscle's fuel. Rather than carbohydrates which tend to promote metabolic waste accumulation. Note, however, that some of these changes include increased capillary (and blood vessel) density and mitochondria, changes that reduce muscle density. Nevertheless, these changes will not cause a significant increase in muscle size.

Since these two goals require quite different methods of training, a good approach may be to periodize your training. That is, train for muscle endurance for 3-4 weeks, and then switch to a training program geared towards building muscle strength.

Q: What is meant by the term Basal Metabolic Rate?

A: Basal Metabolic Rate (BMR) or basal metabolism represents the minimal energy expended to keep a resting, awake body alive. This requires about 60-70% of the total energy use by the body. The processes involved include maintaining a heartbeat, respiration, temperature and other functions. It does not include energy used for physical activity or digesting foods. Basal metabolism accounts for roughly 1 kcalorie/kilogram (2.2 lbs.)/hour. I use the term 'roughly," due to the fact that the amount of energy used for basal metabolism depends primarily upon lean body mass.

Q: What causes delayed onset muscle soreness?

A: The cause for delayed onset muscle soreness (DOMS) has been debated at length by exercise physiologists, and is still not fully understood. Mechanisms for theories proposed in the past have included lactic acid buildup, torn tissue, muscle spasm, and connective tissue damage. Of these, the lactic acid buildup theory, and spasm theory have largely been discounted by exercise physiologists. Currently, the most accepted theory for DOMS seems to be muscle/connective tissue damage due to mechanical forces on the muscle and connective tissue.

Q: I heard that exercising on an empty stomach leads to losses in lean body mass. Should I really be exercising on an empty stomach?

A: There are benefits to working out on an empty stomach, and different benefits when one works out after eating. Ultimately, one should choose the method based on their fitness goals. As a rule of thumb, it may be best to perform workouts on an empty stomach if one's main goal is body fat loss. However, if one is only concerned with gaining lean mass, eating 30-60 minutes before a workout may be a good idea.

For people looking to lose body fat while increasing muscle mass at the same time, it may be best to take advantage of the key benefits of each method. For example, one could try working out on an empty stomach some days, and eat 30-60 minutes before working out on other days (i.e. eat before resistance exercise sessions; do not eat before cardio). Following is a detailed breakdown of the benefits and drawbacks to each method:

Eating 30-60 minutes before a Workout

Benefits:

- Maximizes liver and muscle glycogen, a fuel stored in muscle that is necessary for intense exercise (assuming that the meal is balanced).

- Prevents the breakdown of muscle tissue (by preventing the secretion of the hormone cortisol).

- Allows for longer duration workouts.

- May increase secretion of growth hormone (particularly with exercise that elicits high lactate production, like intense cardio) therefore greater utilization of fat as fuel, free fatty acid (FFA) release, and protein synthesis.

Drawbacks:

- Suppresses FFA release from fat stores (due to the presence of insulin).

- Excess insulin (which easily occurs through eating too many calories or high glycemic foods) may cause hypoglycemia, leading to depleted muscle glycogen stores therefore exerciser "crashes".

Exercise on Empty Stomach

Benefits:

- Increases FFA availability in blood therefore increases the amount fats burned as energy.

- May increase secretion of growth hormone (particularly with exercise that elicits high lactate production, like intense cardio) therefore greater utilization of fat as fuel,

FFA release, and protein synthesis (note that this is an unresolved issue, as it contradicts the bullet above).

Drawbacks:

• Increased production of cortisol therefore leads to the breakdown of muscle tissue.

Q: On certain training days such as when I do back and biceps together, sometimes it is difficult to hold onto the bar because of forearm fatigue. Is there anything I can do to correct this?

A: Forearm strength is often a limiting factor, especially when handling heavy weights vertically such as pull-ups or deadlift. Chalk, sticky pads, or weightlifting straps can help with handling the load when necessary, however, as a rule of thumb, it is best to work through this discomfort since these very activities are some of the best exercises for developing the forearms and building grip strength. On the contrary, straps and chalk should always be used.

When to use straps and chalk:

1. Your ability to hold the weight compromises the safety of the movement, or

2. Lack of grip strength limits your ability to strengthen/develop the target muscle effectively.

Q: I have had a cold the past couple of days and was wondering if it is a good idea to still exercise?

A: You may think it is a good idea not to engage in vigorous exercise when you have the sniffles. However, a new study suggests that if you are well enough to get out of bed, you are probably well enough to get a workout. Researchers at Ball State University in Indiana found that exercising does not delay recovery or worsen symptoms of the common cold.

In the study, 34 moderately fit folks, ages 18-29, were assigned to an exercising group, while 16 additional people of similar age and fitness level were assigned to a non-exercising group. Then both groups were inoculated with a virus to produce upper respiratory illness. The exercising group worked out at 70% of maximum heart rate for 40 minutes per day, every other day.

Researchers collected used facial tissues and administered symptom questionnaires every 12 hours to gauge the progress of the illness and its symptoms. After ten days, analyses of symptoms were similar between the exercising and non-exercising groups. So while you may feel like scaling down your routine if you are feeling under the weather, there seems to be no reason to skip it altogether.

Q: I've heard the terms "concentric and eccentric contractions." What do these mean?

A: A concentric contraction occurs during the lifting phase of an exercise, when the muscle shortens or contracts. For example, when you lift the weight in a bench press, pressing it from your chest to the lock-out position, that is the concentric, or "positive," phase of the exercise. An eccentric contraction occurs during the lowering phase of an exercise, when the muscle lengthens. For example, lowering the weight to your chest during the bench press is the eccentric or "negative," portion of the exercise.

Q: What can I do about 'stretch marks' that appear after I've been weight lifting and gaining size and strength?

A: If you are weight training and gaining some size and muscularity, chances are you will begin to develop stretch marks. This is, to a certain extent, unavoidable. You may minimize their development, however, through the application of a topical antioxidant cream that contains collagen. Regular application of this type of lotion/cream will increase skin elasticity, and thus diminish the formation of stretch marks, but it may not fully prevent their development.

Q: What can I do to prevent muscle cramping?

A: Muscle cramping occurs when a muscle continues to contract, and cannot seem to "let go". The painful sensation one feels is caused by muscle fatigue, and waste products like lactic acid that build up in the muscle. Although the cause of muscle cramps is not entirely understood, a number of factors seem to be involved, including hydration level, electrolyte balance, training history, and chronically tight muscles.

Some factors that may increase muscle cramps:

1. Training history seems to be the most important factor. Exercise beyond an accustomed limit (longer duration, or intensity) will often bring on muscle cramps. However, through regular training, one tends to experience muscle cramps less frequently.

2. Make sure that you are drinking enough water - 10 glasses of water daily (at least 10 oz. each), or if you care to be more precise, 0.6oz/water/lb. of bodyweight. Increase this amount if you consume caffeine. For each cup of coffee, tea, or soda you take in, please be sure to add an additional 10 oz. glass of water for each.

3. Through sweating (especially in a hot environment), one tends to lose electrolytes like sodium, potassium, and magnesium. Normally these are replaced in the diet. However, prolonged exercise (longer than 1 hour) in hot environments may create a need for mineral replenishment. Try adding a bit of salt to your foods, and take a multivitamin/mineral supplement and see if this makes a difference.

4. Lastly, tight muscles are best addressed by stretching before and after every workout. Stretching allows more nutrients, blood, etc. into the muscle, and allows you to dispose of waste materials more easily due to increased blood flow.

Q: What is the current theory on using a weight belt? Should I or shouldn't I use one?

A: Weight belts are a handy tool for helping to protect your back on those lifts that may stress it, but that does not mean you should use them on every lift for every rep. When you do an intense exercise that involves the back, such as squats, it would seem logical that you would want that safety precaution in place at all times.

In doing so, however, you may predispose yourself to an injury by taking the muscles that would ordinarily act as natural back supports out of the equation. Essentially, when you are doing a squat, your primary focus in terms of strength is your leg muscles. What most people don't realize is that you are also simultaneously strengthening your back support muscles; abdominals, lower back, obliques, etc.

When you wear a belt, you take those muscles (to a lesser or greater extent depending upon form) out of the chain, and as such they do not get strengthened to the same degree as do your leg muscles. What this may do in the long run is create an imbalance in the body in terms of overall support and equilibrium, which as you continue to grow stronger and use more weight, may increase the risk of injuring yourself in one way or another.

Perhaps the best way of looking at these muscles is to consider them a chain, and as you know, a chain is only as strong as its weakest link. As such, if you're going to strengthen any part of the chain, you better strengthen the whole chain to keep yourself safe and prevent injuries. When would you want to use a belt? Usually, the only time to use a belt is when you are attempting a maximal lift; anywhere from 4 - 6 reps of a challenging weight that involves back support and all-out effort. At all other times, it's a good idea to simply use good form and have a competent spotter on these exercises.

Q: I have been told all of my life that you have to work out at least 30 to 35 minutes in order to begin burning fat. Is there any scientific data you can provide to prove that the 20-minute aerobic solution does in fact burn fat?

A: When trying to lose body fat, the duration of the workout is less important than total calorie balance (total calories burned). To lose fat, it is necessary to achieve a calorie deficit. That is, the number of calories you burn must be greater than the number of calories you ingest.

Cardiovascular exercise helps you to create this calorie deficit by burning excess calories. Although you can burn calories at any workout intensity, it is most efficient to work at a high-intensity for shorter periods of time compared to long-duration workouts.

For example, working at a high-intensity, one can burn up to 50% more calories in a shorter period of time. More importantly, post workout, you continue to burn calories at an elevated rate up to 142% more than low-intensity aerobics within the first hour following the cardio session. What's more, this elevation in metabolism lasts up to 48 hours post workout, an effect not achieved with low-intensity exercise. The bottom line is that while low-intensity, long-duration exercise is effective for fat loss; typically one sees better results using a high-intensity protocol. Plus, this type of training is more efficient since once spends less time in the gym, but typically experiences better results.

Q: I typically run outdoors, but when it's hot and humid, I head to the treadmill. Does running on the treadmill burn fewer calories?

A: If you're running at speeds under 9 miles an hour (a very fast 6:40-minute-mile pace), treadmill running burns about the same number of calories as running outdoors. But if you run faster than 9 mph, you'll burn fewer calories on the treadmill. The difference can be up to 8 percent because you don't have to overcome wind resistance and because the treadmill belt does propel you along a bit.

Q: A year and a half ago, I started running 5 miles on a treadmill six days a week and lifting weights three times a week. The results have been fabulous; a 74-pound weight loss, a huge drop in blood pressure and an enormous surge in self-esteem. But now my knees ache, especially when I walk downhill. Is this a result of running? What can I do about the pain?

A: Six days a week of high-impact training such as running is very hard on the body, especially the knees. Substituting a low-impact activity such as biking, swimming or the elliptical trainer once or twice a week is much healthier.

Most likely you're experiencing patella-femoral syndrome, also known as pain behind the kneecap. Running, especially on hard surfaces, increases the pressure of the patella (kneecap) on the femur (thighbone) when you bend and straighten your knee.

Q: Is it easier for a man to get six-pack abs than for a woman to?

A: Yes. The appearance of defined, rock-hard ab muscles is possible only if the abs are highly trained and there is very little fat on top of them. On average, women have more total body fat than men, and proportionally they nave more subcutaneous fat. What's more, it's easier for men to lose body fat than it is for women, partly due to hormonal differences. If you put men and women on the same exercise and diet program, men will lose more weight on average. Of course, not every man will lose more fat than every woman will. There are exceptions; some women can achieve a six-pack without tremendous work, and some men have no chance of ever having sleek abs.

The bottom line, don't get frustrated if you can't achieve that six-pack. It may not be a matter of lacking willpower. It could be just a matter of genetic and gender destiny.

Q: I have a friend who does a 5- to 10-minute warm-up on a treadmill, then lifts weights, then does 20 more minutes of cardio. Does her warm-up really count as cardio? I've heard you need to do 15 consecutive minutes to get benefits.

A: A 5- to 10-minute warm-up certainly would count. Since a warm-up is performed at a low intensity, you won't burn as many calories those first few minutes. But that doesn't mean you're not benefiting. Most people don't need more than two or three minutes to get their heart rate up to the lower end of their target zone. At the lower end of the zone — about 60 percent of your maximum heart rate — your body is working hard enough to achieve health and fitness benefits.

There is no research establishing the minimum number of consecutive minutes necessary to "count," but plenty of research has established the benefits of short cardio bouts.

Of course, if you are training for an endurance event such as a 10k or marathon, 10 minute workouts aren't going to cut it. But for general health and fitness you can break it down, research shows tremendous benefits from performing 15 10-minute exercise bouts per week, including cardio exercise, strength training and stretching.

Q: What happens if I go over my target zone for fat burning?

A: You will burn glycogen (blood glucose), which is fine. The problem, however, is that unless you are a highly trained athlete, you don't have high amounts of glycogen stored in your muscles cells and other storage areas. In this case, cortisol, one of the hormones secreted with exercise begins to break down muscle tissue to transform it into glucose so you can continue to exercise/survive. This process is commonly known as "gluconeogenisis," or the new formation of glucose by breaking down muscle.

Q: Why are strong abdominal muscles so important?

A: A strong mid-section will help support the lower back (lumbar spine). It also helps transfer strength and power from the upper body to the lower. In general, the abdominal muscles, lower back, and pelvic region is called the "core." What you need to strive for is "core stability." When the hip flexor muscles are too tight, it causes inflexibility and forward pelvic tilt. Weak abdominals and a tight lower back will create an excessive arch in the lower back known as "sway back." When an imbalance is present in this area, the result can be pain, poor energy transfer in sports, and general body discomfort. Over time, the result can be spinal segments that lip, spur, and even fuse.

Q: How important is massage therapy to an athlete?

A: In one word "VITAL". Massage does the following: reduces stress, decreases recovery time, promotes healing, increases performance, increases speed, releases toxins and it feels oh, so good! Make sure your massage therapist known your tolerance for pain, what type of massage you've experienced, and your intended benefit from the massage.

Q: Should I stretch before or after I work out with weights?

A: Both. Prior to any stretching, a general warm-up should take place. A bike, rower, treadmill or stepper is fine. This is to heat the body's core temperature. Once the core is warm, perform some moderate intensity stretches. Make certain the entire body is stretched, however spend a little extra time on the specific area you intend on training first. After you finish your lifting routine, your body will be very warm and better able to stretch more deeply. This is the time to gently increase the intensity of your stretching.

Q: If I'm very over weight, should I still lift weights? I don't want to bulk up any more.

A: You absolutely should lift weights. It doesn't need to be your focus, but it needs to be included in your complete program. In most cases, weight training is not cardiovascular in nature. This means your body will not use fat as a primary source of energy while lifting weights. However, weight training does make your body better at consuming calories throughout the day. Because a muscle requires more energy to maintain its structure as compared to fat, your body must use (burn) more calories to maintain that muscles integrity. Aside from all this, if you don't maintain or build muscle as you lose weight, you will become what is known as a "thin, fat person." This is a slightly built person who has no muscle mass.

Q: Is there a difference between types of creatines that are currently available?

A: As some people are aware, you can now find creatine on the market in three forms: phosphate, citrate, and monohydrate. My feeling is that the phosphate variety is not easily absorbed by the body and for this reason will not yield effective and substantial results. The citrate variety seemed to be catching on for a time, but again the research is sketchy here. In fact, nearly all the positive clinical studies that have been done on creatine have utilized the monohydrate form, and this is the only form that I currently recommend.

Q: My doctor told me I am allergic to wheat and dairy products. How could this be? Is there a test or a way to really find out if I am allergic?

A: I think the only way you can find this out is by omitting all forms of those foods from your diet for at least a week, then adding the food back and seeing if your symptoms return. Also, since both wheat and dairy products are found in so many foods, you'll have to read the labels of processed foods especially carefully.

Q: I love chocolate. Is it really bad for you? How much can I eat without sabotaging my healthy eating plan?

A: Chocolate isn't all bad. In fact, chocolate is rich in antioxidants called phenolics, the same compounds in red wine that seem to offer protection against heart disease. And cocoa butter, the fat in chocolate, does not appear to be so bad for your heart and arteries. Its principal saturated fat, stearic acid is converted by the body into oleic acid, a heart-healthy monounsaturated fat also found in olive oil. Pick chocolate made with cocoa butter rather than unhealthy fats such as palm and coconut oils. This means look for cocoa to appear in the ingredients before sugar.

Q: I seem to be addicted to sweets. How do you suggest I stop eating foods high in sugar?

A: Taming your sugar cravings could be a matter of slowly reeducating your taste buds or learning to feel satisfied with less. If you slowly cut back on sweets, you will find that healthy sweet foods taste exceptionally sweet - fresh strawberries, frozen grapes, mangoes, dried unsweetened cherries. Treats like these will satisfy your sweet tooth if you take the time to eat them with full attention to taste, aroma, and presentation.

Q: What are the pros and cons of eating farm-raised salmon instead of salmon from the wild? I've heard farmed salmon is not a good source of omega-3 fatty acids because of what the fish are fed.

A: I always choose wild salmon over farmed salmon. Flesh from most pen-raised salmon may be lower in beneficial omega-3 fatty acids and higher in harmful saturated fats than that from their wild cousins - a consequence of what they are fed. And worst of all, is that the under exercised muscles of salmon reared in cages produce a soft, bland-tasting fish that just doesn't stand up to the wild version. The product label will tell you whether or not the fish was farmed.

Q: What is your take on alpha-lipoic acid?

A: Alpha-lipoic acid (ALA) has a number of admirable qualities including the unique ability to work nearly anywhere in the body. It also appears to be safe, readily converts into a useable form, and neutralizes many different kinds of free radicals. This tiny molecule recycles antioxidants such as vitamin C and E, prolonging their effectiveness.

